MW01104682

Seeds of Hope

SEEDS OF HOPE

A PHYSICIAN'S PERSONAL TRIUMPH

OVER PROSTATE CANCER

MICHAEL A. DORSO, M.D.

Acorn Publishing
A Division of Development Initiatives

Seeds of Hope
© 2000 by Michael A. Dorso, M.D.
Acorn Publishing, Division of Development Initiatives
Battle Creek, MI 49016-0084

All rights reserved. This book, or any parts thereof, may not be duplicated in any way without the expressed written consent of its author. The information contained herein is for the personal use of the reader, and may not be incorporated in any commercial programs, other books, databases or any kind of software without the written consent of the publisher or the author. Making copies of this publication, or any portions, for any purpose other than your own, is a violation of United States copyright laws.

Printed in the United States of America
First Edition, 2000

The cover photo is the work of Antonio Vallone and Elizabeth Buie. Elizabeth has photographed Antonio's hands in this powerful image of hope, healing and rebirth living in the seeds he holds. Antonio and Elizabeth are living with prostate cancer. They serve as an inspiration for all those families affected by this illness.
© E. Buie and A. Vallone, Æsthetic Images Photography
www.aesthetic-images.com

The images used herein were obtained from IMSI's Master Collection. 1895 Francisco Blvd. East, San Rafael, CA 94901-5506, USA

Library of Congress Cataloging-in-Publication Data

Dorso, Michael A. (Michael Anthony), 1942-
  Seeds of hope : a physician's personal triumph over prostate cancer /
by Michael A. Dorso ; edited by Doreen L. Skardarasy.-- 1st ed.
    p. cm.
Includes bibliographical references (p.   ).
  ISBN 0-9678801-6-5
  1. Dorso, Michael A. (Michael Anthony), 1942---Health. 2.
Prostate--Cancer--Patients--California--Biography. 3.
Emergency physicians--California--Biography. I. Skardarasy,
Doreen L. (Doreen Lyn), 1949- II. Title.
  RC280.P7 D67 2000
  362.1'9699463'0092--dc21

                                                    00-010024

ISBN 0-9678801-6-5

Dedication

This book is lovingly dedicated
to my wife, Sherry
And to our four children
Tammy
Amy
Jeffrey
Elizabeth

They were a source of strength,
And a prime reason
I had to beat this disease!

ATTENTION READERS

Disclaimer

This book is intended as an attempt to share the author's experiences with prostate cancer. It should not be construed as medical advice, nor as a medical opinion about any reader's personal medical condition. It is sold with the understanding that the publisher and author are not engaged in the practice of medicine with this book.

It is not the purpose of this book to reprint all the medical information that is available, nor to outline all the therapeutic choices available for a patient with prostate cancer, but to complement, amplify, and supplement other texts. You are encouraged to read all the available material, learn as much as possible about prostate cancer, and to tailor the information to your individual needs. Cancer therapy as outlined in this book is not a cure-all, and is not for everyone. A man with prostate cancer, or any other illness, should never make a therapeutic decision without consulting his own physician.

Every effort has been made to make this book as accurate as possible. However, there may be mistakes both typographical and in content. The purpose of this book is to educate and entertain. The author and Acorn Publishing shall have neither liability nor responsibility to any person or entity with respect to any loss or damage caused, or alleged to be caused, directly or indirectly by the information contained in this book. Furthermore, this book contains information on prostate cancer only up to the publishing date.

If you do not wish to be bound by the above, you may return this book to the publisher for a full refund.

CONTENTS

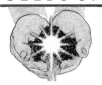

INTRODUCTION

"You have cancer." This short sentence will crash into any conversation with the force of a falling airliner! No, that's not nearly formidable enough. Cancer is a nuclear bomb—suddenly found ticking in the middle of your life. Only God knows when it will reach critical mass.

As a physician, I often have to break bad news to patients. Increasingly the bad news is prostate cancer. There just is no tactful way to tell a man that he has prostate cancer. How do I tell a man that an alien presence has taken residence in his loins, an alien presence that may burst out of his pelvis at any time to destroy him—despite medicine's best efforts?

I heard the bad news myself three years ago. A colleague told me that I had prostate cancer. With those words my life was forever changed. I was launched on a tumultuous voyage of discovery through which I am still sailing.

What does a physician do when he has cancer? Men have phoned me from all over the country—men with recently diagnosed prostate cancer—eager to know the answer to that question. In counseling these men, still reeling from their bad news, I've been able to speak as both physician and patient. I understood their shock, angst, fear, anger, and denial. I've been there.

During these compelling conversations, I came to realize that a man's very survival depends on his positive attitude. I remember men reacting with disbelief, when I suggested that cancer could bear a gift in its hands—that cancer could actually bring a healing influence into a person's life. During one of these dialogues, I realized I had to write this book.

One hundred and eighty thousand American men will discover they have prostate cancer every year. Each one of these men will feel enormous pressure to choose his therapy quickly. He will be expected to make his life or death decision with little knowledge of his options—or their consequences. Worse yet, he will find the medical community in disarray. If he's at all perceptive, he'll realize that there is no consensus among his physicians. There is no freeway through Cancerland. He'll have to carefully pick his own path.

That path could be surgical, or non-surgical. It could include radiation therapy of various types (including radioactive implants), hormonal suppression, dietary changes, freezing the cancer with cold probes, cooking the cancer with microwaves, or watchful waiting. Alternative medicine offers an even wider array of choices. I chose a non-surgical path. For me this was the right decision. In these chapters, I make my case for that decision.

The past three years were among the most dynamic of my life. I certainly was never bored. It was one hell of a ride! My tale shares the joys, fears, triumphs, frustrations, and growth I experienced as I found my path through cancer's dense undergrowth.

Seeds of Hope is for those one hundred and eighty thousand men and their families. Here is my story of prostate cancer. I will take you through the dragon's belly with me. Be forewarned: "The way out of the dragon's belly is rarely exhilarating, but the struggle can be magnificent—in retrospect."

Michael A. Dorso, M.D.

ABOUT THE AUTHOR

Dr. Michael Dorso earned his Bachelor's degree in physics at the University of Florida before beginning medical studies at the University of Miami. He earned his Doctor of Medicine in 1969, and began a ten-year career as a flight surgeon in the USAF. His military career included a tour of duty with The Strategic Air Command, as Chief of Flight Medicine at Plattsburg AFB. He served in Saudi Arabia as an advisor to the Royal Saudi Air Force, before finishing his distinguished career at Edwards AFB as director of Aerospace Medicine.

He continued his career in Aerospace Medicine as a civilian, at NASA's Dryden Flight Research Center. There he participated in flight testing the Space Shuttle for three years.

In 1979 Dr. Dorso returned to his first love, Emergency Medicine. Presently residing in northern California with his wife and children, he serves as an emergency physician in a busy community hospital.

Early in his career, Dr. Dorso grasped the importance of a positive attitude in healing. His daily interactions with all manner of patients brought him to a carefully reasoned philosophy of life and its illnesses—illnesses which ultimately affect us all. He saw how important it was for a patient to assume responsibility for his own therapy. He realized that patients with a spiritual concept of life fare better. He began planning a book advocating those philosophical principles.

Dr. Dorso was diagnosed with prostate cancer on a routine physical exam three years ago. That diagnosis was a life-altering event. In his search for information and perspective, he saw a desperate need for an informative, personal book about prostate cancer. His book, *Seeds of Hope: A Physician's Personal Triumph Over Prostate Cancer*, addresses that need. This book tells the engaging tale of Dr. Dorso's own illness in the context of his philosophy. It is written for men with prostate cancer and the families who love them.

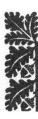

CHAPTER 1

CANCER! ME?

"Mike, unless you want to spend the next week in this cave, we'd better get out of here fast!" Everett was right. A winter storm was threatening to bury us in our retreat. If we stayed at this altitude, we would be snowbound. We had to get to safety.

The day had started well enough, with a glorious hike in the High Sierra! I did not suspect what surprises it held for me that afternoon. My friend Everett and I had climbed to a cave we'd spotted on a cliff face. The climb had been an arduous snowshoe scramble above Carson Pass. Standing triumphant at the cave's mouth, we watched an early winter storm begin to swirl about us. Everett grinned at me, and in his best T.V. commercial voice said: "Guys, it just doesn't get any better than this." I stood there feeling the cold wind on my face, and silently agreed. We still had what it took to conquer this mountain! I rejoiced in our virility.

Watching the storm gather its clouds about our mountain sanctuary, we shared our lunch in the shelter of the cave's mouth. The sky was soon glowering, and the wind had developed a menacing sound echoing against the cave walls. We knew a storm was due that night, but this one seemed eager to get down to business. Everett walked to the threshold of the cave and was staggered by the wind! He looked alarmed as he returned to retrieve his coat. I agreed: We had to cut the hike short. Reluctantly we headed home early. At least the hike out was downhill, and the wind to our backs.

On the drive home, we stopped at a ski lodge for coffee and blackberry pie—a reward for our hard day's hiking. After we ordered our pie, Everett excused himself to wash up. Alone with my thoughts, I remembered that I might be harboring a cancer. I wondered how much longer I would be hiking these mountain trails. I had undergone a biopsy of my prostate gland a week earlier, and dreaded the news. The report might be available today. Why not phone my urologist, and get this worry off my back? It would certainly be worth the cost of a long distance call! A few minutes later I had Nicholas Simopoulos, M.D. on the phone.

I will forever remember that brief conversation. Even over the phone I could tell that Nick was uncomfortable as he spoke. His words were agonizingly slow to appear, and I intuitively knew from his tone that the news was not going to be good.

"Mike, I'm afraid that I have some bad news. We found malignant cells in your prostate gland. We're going to have to remove your prostate." He paused awkwardly and then said: "Why don't you come in to see me this week, and we'll talk about it?"

I couldn't believe what I was hearing! **Malignant? Me? Remove my prostate**? I could tell that Nick was uncomfortable discussing things of such import over the phone, but I wasn't ready to hang up. Trying to find some sanity here, I asked, "You mean a prostatectomy? What are the complications?"

Nick's answer was painfully blunt, **"fifty percent impotency, and three percent urinary incontinence."**

I couldn't believe this was happening! My mind began to rebel, refusing to deal with this news. Feeling stunned and nauseated, I hung up after muttering something vaguely like: "Thanks, I'll give you a call."

I don't know how long I stood there by the phone, trying to comprehend what was happening to me. I wondered how often Nick had to tell a man that he had cancer. The "fifty percent, three percent" figures seemed to roll off his tongue before I even finished the question. I could tell that he'd answered that one a few times. I sensed the irony in this scene: **Michael A. Dorso, M.D. has just become Michael A. Dorso, PATIENT!**

In the natural order of things, I was the one who delivered the bad news. How many times have I told a man that he might soon die? Suddenly it was my turn. I sensed that I had just crossed a major threshold in my life. I had just been pushed over that line demarcating the doctor-patient relationship. Somehow I found myself on the wrong side. I was forevermore to be counted among the seriously ill.

This seemed to come out of nowhere! I had always figured that the big event was going to be a heart attack. All the men in my family had died of heart disease. Wait a minute! Dad had dealt with prostate cancer two years

ago! I shouldn't have been so surprised. I grinned sardon-
ically at the macabre thought:

"At least I won't be pestered ever again by life insurance salesmen."

I thought about Everett back at the table with the
melting pies a-la-mode. What was I to say to him? How
does one announce that he has cancer? Did I want to tell
him? Did I even want to tell anyone? I had heard stories
of people experiencing discrimination because of their
cancer. I remembered that cancer patients were not
allowed to donate blood. I knew there was a great deal of
ignorance out there. I had even encountered people who
considered cancer to be contagious. Prostate cancer is
especially suspect because of its intimate connection to
one's sexuality. If it wasn't contagious, might it be God's
punishment for sexual indiscretion? Maybe a virus spread
by a promiscuous life? Many people just seemed uncomfortable with cancer patients. Did I really want to just leap
into this marked change in social status without a bit of
solitary reflection? I had to think fast as I walked back to
the table.

Everett's face was flushed red from the cold wind
we'd endured that day. He looked strong and vibrant. He
was still enjoying the aura of our adventure—two middle
aged men still able to snowshoe a mile and a half high!
We had rejoiced in our masculinity and strength, both
secretly hoping that we might have been snowed into that
cave. Still not too old for excitement. Still able to dream
about adventure. Everett had become one of my closest

friends. We had shared many an intimate thought over the years. Now I sensed a chasm between us. He dwelled in the kingdom of the healthy. I had somehow fallen to a different realm.

Everett knew me well enough to see that I was distracted by my thoughts. It was obvious that he wanted to hear the news, but he is a patient man. We sat and ate our pie quietly for a few moments. I decided to share the bad news, I just wasn't sure how to broach the subject. I was surprised by how embarrassed I felt!

Everett's patience finally ended. "So what did the doctor say?"

I just blurted out, *"I have prostate cancer."*

There it was again, that powerful sense of embarrassment! So this is how it feels to tell someone you have cancer! I had just admitted that I was somehow gravely flawed. I felt personally responsible for my new diagnosis. I saw the shock on Everett's face and sensed the unspoken question: "How can this happen?"

I asked myself the same question. For me there had always been a sense of order in the medical world. Life was divided into two camps: **"The Sick"**—we called them patients—and **"The Caregivers."** As a physician, I enjoyed privileges of only the highest ranks of Caregivers. I even had a designated parking space at the hospital attesting to my status. As a Caregiver, I managed very nicely to distance myself from human frailties. Here I was fifty-four years old and had never been seriously ill. (OK. I had my tonsils removed at age seven.)

There is a popular mantra that sounds something like this: If you don't smoke or drink, if you exercise regularly, and if you take care of yourself, you can live to a ripe old age and enjoy those golden years. Anyone who becomes ill usually violates the mantra. It had been a great defense mechanism.

There is a temptation among Caregivers to blame the patient for his illness: "No wonder he has coronary artery disease. Look at the way he overeats!...I'll bet his cholesterol is off the charts. He's fat and sedentary." And so goes the chant. The emphysema patient smokes too much. The drug addict is somehow weak-willed. The ulcer patient worries or drinks too much. Occasionally, there is the poor unfortunate who was simply born with PPP (Piss Poor Protoplasm). Can't hold him or her responsible. Otherwise, being among **"The Sick"** carries the onus of personal responsibility. I began to understand my embarrassment.

I suddenly realized the danger in such a mantra. We all someday succumb to a fatal illness. It's part of the human condition to eventually decline and die—except now it becomes our fault! Perhaps no-fault illness would be the next corrective concept to take its place beside no-fault insurance and no-fault divorce.

We finished our pie in silence. Everett is a priest, with considerable experience in counseling people. He was astute enough to know that I needed time to process this shocking news. Any meaningful conversation would have to come from me. As for me, I was so stunned that I was having difficulty concentrating. My thoughts were chaotic. I knew I should be formulating a plan of action, but I had no idea where to start! The final product was silence.

We did have a good conversation during the two-hour drive home. I finally opened up and spilled my guts. Was it mere coincidence that put me in the company of my priest at this time of crisis? I knew I had a great deal to learn about cancer. I had plenty to learn about illness and dying. I didn't realize how much I would learn about living.

Cancer had been a topic of medicine that held little interest for me. Even as a medical student I somehow found it abhorrent. It conjured up memories of losing battles with an invisible enemy that took no prisoners. I can still recall skeletal patients too weak to get out of bed; bald women on chemotherapy vomiting incessantly; men with bloody diarrhea and bloated abdomens; others slowly suffocating with lung cancer. I had seen terribly disfiguring surgery as physicians attempted to cut out the affliction. I had witnessed the consequences of radiation therapy as radiotherapists desperately tried to burn it out. Why any physician would choose cancer as a life's work remained a puzzlement for me.

As an Emergency Physician, I was schooled in the clinical complications of various cancers. I had seen elderly men with prostate cancers unable to urinate. The cancer had obstructed their bladders or damaged their kidneys. I knew that the end stage of prostate cancer was a difficult death. I was damn sure I didn't want to die that way. I realized that strength would come with knowledge and vowed to be in the library the next morning.

Meanwhile I had to decide how I was going to tell my family about my cancer. Sherry has been my wife for more than three decades. We've been through a lot together, but most of the medical focus had been on her: bearing children, hysterectomy, and breast biopsies. I had managed to stay away from doctors and their nostrums. I didn't relish my turn under the spotlight.

I recalled the slogan: "When a person gets cancer, the whole family gets cancer." I didn't want this illness to devastate my vibrant, loving, and active family. I knew that my reaction was going to set the pace for Sherry and our four adult children. I needed to break the news with honesty and optimism, without minimizing the seriousness of our situation.

I returned home that evening resolved to do this right. A private conversation with Sherry was the right place to start, but it would have to wait. Sherry had prepared our family supper. Throughout the meal I harbored the news, feeling less than genuine keeping such important news from everyone. The dinner conversation seemed unimportant. I claimed fatigue from my day's hiking and allowed myself to remain silent through the meal.

I felt separated from my loved ones—a separation that could be unhealthy if allowed to continue. I began to understand how important it would be to stay involved with my family and friends. It was then I made one of my first decisions: I would not be isolated by this illness! There was no way I could withhold this news from my expanding circles of family, friends, and co-workers. I would have to tell everyone—Sherry first.

I quietly asked Sherry to join me in our room. We sat on the bed and held hands. I could see the concern growing on her face. I felt awkward. I had to speak quickly before she became alarmed.

"Sherry, I called Nick today. The news isn't good. My biopsy is positive. He said I have prostate cancer."

Amazing woman—she didn't even flinch! "So what does it mean?"

"I don't really know yet. I'll probably be facing surgery or radiation therapy. Nick told me that there was a big chance that I could be impotent—maybe fifty percent. I guess I'll be out of work for a while, recovering from surgery. I could end up with trouble peeing for the rest of my life."

Sherry looked in my eyes as she asked, "Are you OK?"

"Frankly, I'm pretty scared!"

I admitted that I was scared! That was probably the first time, in thirty-four years of marriage, that I told

Sherry *I was scared*. That confession was profoundly cathartic! My voice was breaking, and tears welled in my eyes. We held each other—and wept. I could feel a wave of fear threatening to wash over me. There were so many questions: Would our finances hold together, if I didn't do well? Would I be in pain? Disfigured?

I buried my face in my wife's bosom, trying to somehow find strength and courage to face what might lie ahead. I hungered for the security of my childhood. I wanted someone to tell me that this was all a mistake, that all would be well.

Sherry was the first to speak again. "What are we going to tell the children?"

I managed to lift my head and pull things together a bit.

"I really don't know. Stalling seems like a good idea for now. I think we should know what I'm going to do before we break the news."

We agreed to inform our offspring, once I had a plan of action. I gave Sherry a major league hug and left her sitting on the bed. Her face, her posture were unmistakable: she had been stunned by the news.

As for me, I just couldn't stand any more emotion! I needed a break. I needed purposeful activity. I headed for the computer with a plan to search the Internet for information. Crummy idea! My refuge at the computer would not be for long. My eldest daughter, Tammy, stormed into the study and verbally accosted me.

"Dad, what the hell is going on? You sit glumly

through supper, then drag Mother into your room with the door closed. Thirty minutes later she appears with red, swollen eyes, and you're hiding in the study!"

So much for stalling! We had to deal with this now. No time for planning. John Lennon was so right when he said, "Life is what happens to you while you're making plans." I took Tammy into Beth's room, invited Sherry to join us, and broke the news again. I tried to put a positive spin on events. "I had good doctors; We found it early; I planned to be cured." They took it all in with admirable courage. It wouldn't be the last time I was impressed with the resiliency of my children.

My only son, Jeffrey, was attending the University of Cairo on a study exchange program. I took time to write a long letter to him that evening. My daughter Amy was living across town. I called her and broke the news.

As I hung up, I was exhausted. I barely had enough energy for my bedtime rituals of showering and brushing. In bed, Sherry and I held each other. As I drifted off to sleep in the comfort of her embrace, I wondered what this would mean for our sexuality. I suspected that our love life was soon to change, but I didn't have energy to think about that now.

Chapter 2

Pappy Yokum Had a Prostrate Gland.

As a young man I enjoyed the Little Abner comic strip. I especially enjoyed Sadie Hawkins Day, which happened every leap year. On Sadie Hawkins Day the women were allowed to chase the men. The bachelors got a running head start. What followed was a scene reminiscent of the Oregon Land Rush. The brides-to-be would be off in hot pursuit. Any captured man had to marry his captor. He was typically carried back to the starting line over his new bride's shoulder and greeted by the minister.

I was especially delighted by Mammy and Pappy Yokum. Mammy Yokum was a tough, no-nonsense, pipe-smoking, good-hearted matriarch. Pappy was a diminutive, sweet fellow with a cute potbelly who could never hurt a fly. One day Pappy suffered a blow to the head and became a regular Mr. Hyde. I watched in amusement as Pappy went about performing various dastardly deeds through a week of comic strips. Mammy finally took him to the doctor, who x-rayed Pappy's head. The doc was triumphant as he displayed the film on his view box.

"Ah-Ha! Here is the problem!"

The x-ray showed Pappy's skull with a little gland in the center—shaped vaguely like Pappy, complete with potbelly. Unfortunately the gland was lying on its back. It had been knocked over—prostrate—at the base of Pappy's skull.

The doctor explained: "Pappy's upright gland has been knocked prostrate. Pappy Yokum has a 'prostrate gland'!"

Unfortunately, there didn't seem to be much Doc could do about the problem, and Pappy went back to his nefarious ways for another week of comics. Finally, in exasperation Mammy KO'd Pappy with a true round-house punch. He awoke once again his usual sweet, upright self. A repeat x-ray showed—you guessed it—his prostrate gland once again in the upright position.

I hate to admit it, but this was my concept of a prostate gland through most of college—complete with the misspelling as "prostrate." One day I visited a friend, Bill, who was in pre-med school. Bill greeted me with the standard, "How ya doin'?" I cleverly announced that I wasn't feeling so well, and "Perhaps I had a prostrate gland." Bill looked perplexed and said, "I sure hope you do!"

Suddenly sensing that I was displaying gross igno-rance, I quickly changed the topic of conversation. That evening I borrowed a fraternity brother's anatomy book. Damned if I didn't find a real prostate gland! I had no idea there was such a thing in my groin.

There are times in my practice of medicine when I am dumbfounded by patients' ignorance of their bodies. I then harken back to this story to regain perspective of what my body awareness was like, before I spent eight years in formal medical education.

———◂••••••••▸———

So what exactly is the prostate gland? What does it do? What's the big deal?

The prostate gland is a plum-sized organ seated below the urinary bladder. It produces about eighty percent of the fluid in a man's semen. That obviously makes it important for reproduction, but that's not the big deal.

The big deal is that it actually is wrapped around the urethra. (That's the tubing running from the bladder and out the penis.) It doesn't take a rocket scientist to realize that any disease or tinkering with the gland runs the risk of obstructing a man's flow of urine, and then he can't pee. And that's just the first problem.

The nerves responsible for a man's erection are embedded in the surface of the prostate gland. Damage those nerves during therapy, and a man becomes impotent. Now he can't perform sexually. That's two.

Any surgery to remove the prostate gland can injure the nerves and muscles controlling the release of urine— rendering a man incontinent of urine. Now he's dribbling and wearing diapers. That's three!

———◂••••••••▸———

Our society doesn't seem to take prostate problems seriously. I confess, I have been one of the worst offenders. I received one of my favorite birthday cards when I turned fifty. It was hand made by a friend with a cartoon of a little old man sitting on a commode. The inscription read:

> *Two basic rules for men over fifty:*
> ❶ *Never pass a urinal.*
> ❷ *Never ignore an erection.*

The image of an old man having trouble with his bodily functions somehow seemed a bit funny. I confess that I've told and retold that joke many a time. Now I'm beginning to believe in instant karma.

While Pappy Yokum's 'prostrate' gland may be laughable, prostate cancer is not. If you like to think in round numbers, here are a few. About 180,000 American men are told they have prostate cancer each year. About 32,000 men die every year because of their cancers. About the same number of women die annually of breast cancer. Approximately the same number of men and women die from AIDS. Given the public outcry over AIDS, and the publicity afforded breast cancer, it's easy to see that prostate cancer truly is a silent epidemic.

Let's just stop and look at these numbers. The annual number of men diagnosed with prostate cancer is about six times the number dying of their disease. The odds are about the same as Russian Roulette, which means that most men with prostate cancer are dying of something else! They are dying with their prostate cancer—not of their cancer. How can that be?

These odds make sense when you learn that most of these are older men. They are also subject to all the other illnesses of mankind. For example, let's not forget that heart disease is still the greatest killer in this country—especially among older men. It's very possible to have prostate cancer and die of a heart attack—or get run over by the proverbial Mack truck.

Medical advances have doubled the early diagnoses of prostate cancer since 1978. This has created a flurry of activity, resembling an epidemic. I suspect that the pace will continue to quicken. The huge cohort of Baby-Boomer men are crossing over age fifty. The "Boomers" are a demographic force that has transformed every aspect of American society, as they have passed through their generational rites of passage. The Baby Boom is soon to become the Geezer Boom. Just wait until they discover their prostate glands! I have no doubt that these men will bring new energy and finances to the world of prostate cancer. I've noticed that the mainstream press is already discovering prostate cancer.

Prostate cancer is not an equal opportunity disease! It's a disease of men only—primarily older men, although younger men in their 50's, 40's, and even 30's are not beyond its reach. African-American men have a higher incidence of the disease and possibly a more malignant course. Farmers are at greater risk. (Perhaps due to exposure to agricultural chemicals?) This is a cancer that runs in families. A man whose father had prostate cancer has to be more vigilant. With these few exceptions, prostate cancer crosses all races and class structures. It does not respect fame, wealth, religion, or power.

A listing of men touched by this disease includes such diverse religious leaders as the Ayatollah Khomeini, Rev. Lewis Farrakhan, and South African Bishop Desmond Tutu. Dr. Linus Pauling won two Nobel Prizes, popularized the use of vitamin C for colds, and succumbed to the disease. Entertainment icons with prostate cancer include Jerry Lewis, Don Ameche, Sean Connery, Frank Zappa, Robert Goulet, Ed Asner, and Sidney Poitier. Other prominent people include Bob Dole, General H. Norman Schwarzkopff (both had prostatectomies), David Brinkley, Jesse Helms, Charleton Heston (Moses), and Rudy Giuliani. Athletic ability offers no protection. Arnold Palmer, Stan Musial, Bobby Riggs, Johnny Unitas, and Richard Petty have all suffered with it. Joe Torre managed the Yankees to World Series championships twice in his first three seasons with the team, and was stricken with prostate cancer at age fifty-eight. International figures include Charles de Gaulle, Francois Mitterand, (both men aggressively suppressed the news for years), King Hussein of Jordan, and Moshe Arens.

The average American is 65 years old at diagnosis. We don't hear much about prostate cancer from the third world countries where the average life span is about 45 years. They just don't live long enough! At autopsy many men are found to have unsuspected prostate cancer—men who have died of other, unrelated causes. Some studies suggest that 40% of men over age 50 have microscopic prostate cancer, or worse. I once heard a pathologist conjecture that most men would develop prostate cancer if they just lived long enough.

Prostate cancer is usually a slow growing malignancy. Despite the fact that many of the above-mentioned men died of their cancer, a diagnosis of prostate cancer is not an immediate death sentence. Depending on several variables, untreated prostate cancer may take ten years to end a man's life.

Given that fact, an elderly man with other severe illnesses would probably avoid aggressive therapy. In such a case, most physicians would recommend close observation and treatment of complications as they arose. "Watchful Waiting" is the cautious term used here. It's an accepted plan for managing prostate cancer.

———⋘•●●●●●⋙———

I was fifty-four years old, and I had prostate cancer. In the world of prostate cancer I was a pediatric patient! As one friend said so indelicately, "Assuming you plan to live a normal life span, this cancer has plenty of time to kill you!" If I was planning to live another thirty years, I had to find a way to kill this beast and make sure it stayed dead!

I knew that I was in a unique position to research my disease and participate in my treatment. As a physician schooled in medical terminology, I could make sense of the gobbledygook in medical literature. Furthermore, I was determined to educate myself and take responsibility for my therapy. With that determination, I headed for the medical library at my first opportunity.

I decided to start with a basic textbook on urological surgery. If I was facing a possible prostatectomy, I wanted to see what the surgery entailed. The drawings I found were beautifully illustrated. They depicted a man under anesthesia with a huge incision starting at the upper abdomen, moving down and around the belly button, and extending all the way down to the pubic bone. Good Lord! Why did it have to be such a huge cut?

A surgeon was cutting away the prostate gland. He severed the urethra at the top and bottom of the prostate gland, and lifted the gland from its bed. The next illustration showed the gaping urethra protruding from the bottom of the bladder, while the other end rose from the pelvis—inches apart. The surgeon pulled down the urethra and bladder until the severed ends met and then sewed them together.

I began to feel nauseated and anxious. Normally such pictures of surgery were not very disturbing, because I imagined myself the surgeon. Suddenly I was the patient! It was me lying there with my viscera exposed! It reminded me of the map at the mall: a big orange arrow pointing at my groin, flashing, "You Are Here!"

My heart began pounding as I read on. The surgery was labeled a "Radical Prostatectomy." Radical! Why did my colleagues choose such ominous nomenclature? Was Nick planning a radical prostatectomy? On ME? In a radical prostatectomy the surgeon removes the prostate gland, the seminal vesicles, and the neighboring lymph glands. That makes it "radical." The seminal vesicles lie behind the prostate and store the sperm cells. Because of their intimate plumbing with the prostate gland, the cancer can easily spread there. They have to go too.

Eventually the cancer spreads to the lymph glands nearest the prostate gland. During surgery, before the prostate gland is removed, the surgeon removes any suspicious looking lymph glands, and rushes them to the waiting pathologist, who does a quick analysis. He's looking for cancer in the lymph glands. If he finds cancer, it's too late for a surgical cure. The surgery usually stops there.

I had to stop there. I truly was becoming ill. How the hell had I found myself in this bear trap! Yes, trapped! As surely as if my leg were writhing in the steel teeth of a fur trapper! I could feel panic rising! I was overwhelmed with an irrational urge to run and hide, but there would be no running. I was carrying this killer with me. In a scene reminiscent of the movie *Alien*, I had a monster in the very core of my body—a monster that threatened to burst out of my pelvis at any time and destroy me.

As I drove home the nausea persisted. I began to feel suffocated! I was breathing harder, faster. I opened a window. The wind in my face seemed to help a bit. I had to get myself together. I was scheduled to work an evening shift that night. I pulled off the highway and stopped at a favorite spot by the lake. Walking alone on the shore had always proven therapeutic for my soul. I had to get my thoughts in order—had to make some sense of this. As I sat on a large rock overlooking the water, I n to pray.

But I didn't know what to say to my God! The words wouldn't come. Was I going to beg Him to take away this illness? I had an image of billions of souls on earth all repetitiously begging for favors. Every soul with a serious illness praying for a cure, for a miracle. What a horrific cacophony that must be—even to a God!

I thought of The Lord's Prayer. "*Thy will be done, on earth as it is in heaven.*" Was this cancer the will of my God? Is everything that happens on this planet the absolute will of God? Would a perfect God create a world so rife with imperfection, so filled with disease? I remember asking my mother why God created mosquitoes—as she was smearing calamine lotion on my bites. She paused for a minute and then replied, "No, I think someone else made the mosquitoes." That was my first real comprehension that there may be sinister forces afoot.

I rejected the thought that this cancer was the work of evil forces. Likewise, I couldn't accept that this was just random bad luck. It had to have significance, even if it was simply another manifestation of humanity's fall from grace. I quietly suspected that I had agreed to this before I was even born. I knew this cancer had a spiritual significance. If so, then it was my responsibility to understand the lesson to be learned here. I remembered what Richard Bach said in his moving book *Illusions*:

"There is no such thing as a problem without a gift for you in its hands.

You seek problems because you need their gifts."

It was hard for me to imagine that there could be any gift in the hands of cancer, but I was willing to consider it.

———◦•◦••••◦•◦———

I have a friend, Lee Sturgeon Day, who has survived breast cancer. Her book *A Slice of Life* chronicles her path to health through alternative therapies. She is a unique lady who saw spiritual significance in her cancer and expressed it eloquently. She actually speaks of healing one's life through cancer:

> This sense of the human being in a continual creative development is very important to me. I already accepted that my cancer was a final expression in my body of a long process of dis-ease in body, soul, and spirit that had been proceeding for many years before attaining a physical form. The lumps and bumps were a cry for help, a cry for change. I also saw it as a challenge. (One I would gladly do without in these first days, but a challenge nonetheless.) And if I survived, I hoped to get better in the sense of being better than I was before. Though I quaked at the thought of dying, and prayed that some voice from heaven would quickly assure me that I would not, I wanted to make something out of this illness, or allow it to make something out of me; to bring me to greater wholeness, a deeper sense of myself and the world...If we do not develop, the illness is wasted...Development is also emphatically not seen only in the context of a surviving life. We may be healed in some much more significant way, even though we die.

I grasped that this was to be one of my life's trials—perhaps even a last one. I recognized that this cancer was to be my path of development—hopefully a healing path! I was actually encouraged by the thought that a horrid disease could be a source of healing. This was going to take some serious praying. It had been a long time since I really prayed. I smiled to myself. It looked like my "development" had already begun.

No, I wasn't going to ask my God to take this cup from me. What I needed was His grace of understanding. That would be my prayer. I would add a second prayer: *God grant me the strength to endure with dignity what lay ahead.*

CHAPTER 3

LET'S START AT THE BEGINNING.

certitude

I had always enjoyed robust health. My last physical exam had been in the US Air Force over twenty years ago. I was grateful for my good health—grateful for my status as a Caretaker. I didn't need a physical exam. I was a physician. It was my job to know when someone was ill. I obviously wasn't ill. That egoism could have cost me my life.

Fortunately our group of physicians changed medical insurance plans to save money. Yes, even physicians are trying to find ways to reduce the personal cost of health care! I was now listed as a patient with a Health Maintenance Organization (HMO). I needed to pick a "primary care doctor" who would oversee my medical care. Muttering that this was a waste of time, I looked over the list of available physicians. I was pleased to see Bradley Barnhill, M.D. on the list. Bradley is a young internist, a few years out of his training. When I first met him at work, I couldn't get over how young he appeared. In fact I've noticed that all the new docs are looking mighty young these days. I had worked with Bradley to rescue critically ill patients over the past few years, and I liked his style. I decided that he would be my man. When I called him, he was chagrined to hear that I had not had

25

*y*sical exam in twenty years. He suggested that I
*n*edule one.

⸺⟨●●●●●⟩⸺

And so the first week of May found me waiting in
Bradley's examination room. I was bemused by my hairy
legs, protruding from the bottom of my gown. It was my
first realization of how cold I could feel in a room with
only a thin paper gown to ward off the elements. I was
especially struck with how vulnerable I felt when I gave
up my clothes. His nurse warned me that this would be a
"complete exam"—code word for rectal exam—so everything had to come off.

The rectal exam has to be one of the most embarrassing things we doctors do to our patients.
Unfortunately it is the only way to palpate a patient's
prostate gland (and other organs such as an inflamed
appendix). It can be a lifesaver if the physician feels an
early rectal or prostate cancer. Reluctant medical students
are repeatedly reminded to do the right thing and examine
their patients backside. Their work is considered incom-
plete, if they leave out the rectal exam. No patient enjoys
having a physician put a gloved finger into his or her
rectum. It's embarrassing and uncomfortable for both the
physician and patient. And now I was to be once again
reminded that I was on the other side of the patient-doctor
relationship.

⸺⟨●●●●●⟩⸺

My first prostate exam had been for an Air Force
physical at age twenty-one. I was one of twenty-five

recruits being poked and probed that day. At one point I was sent into a small room for my digital rectal examination. The doctor was there with a box of new gloves on the right and a wastebasket overflowing with used gloves on the left. He instructed me: "Bend over and spread your cheeks." I dutifully did as commanded while he stuck his gloved finger in my rectum. Imagine spending half your life in school so you can do that all day long! I remember wondering whom he had pissed off to get that job!

Doctor Bradley Barnhill was a thorough man. He performed a careful, head to toes, physical exam. I wondered: "Is he always this thorough with all his patients?" We were both aware that there were two physicians in the room—one very personally committed to the process. The digital rectal exam was uncomfortable, but tolerable.

Bradley reassured me: "Everything seems in order. Your prostate gland felt normal. You're lucky. You're a healthy man. Now, I'd like you to stop by the lab for some routine blood tests."

Wanting to be a good patient, I did as I was told. I gave my blood to the vampires living among the test tubes in the lab, and went home feeling good. The universe was unfolding exactly as it should. I had many of these blood tests informally in the past, and they had always been normal. I anticipated another confirmation of my good health the next day.

The Fates had other plans.

Bradley called me the next day and told me that all the tests were normal except for one called Prostate Specific Antigen (PSA). I didn't even realize that he had ordered a PSA level. I knew the PSA was a blood test for prostate cancer. I was aware that there was controversy swirling about it—some doubts about its reliability. Arguments were raging in the medical literature about making it part of the routine exam for every man over fifty. My father's prostate cancer had been found on such a routine blood test. I had otherwise paid little attention to PSA testing.

Quite frankly, it was out of my scope of practice. I'm an emergency physician. When I'm caring for a man injured in a violent rollover car crash, his PSA is not the first thing on my mind! I'd be willing to bet that the words "PSA" have never been uttered on the television drama E.R.

Trying to sound casual I asked Bradley: "So what was the number?" He told me it was 10.4. I didn't even know what was supposed to be a normal number.

"How bad is that?" I asked.

Bradley explained that a normal PSA value is less than 4, but was quick to add that many things could artificially elevate the PSA, including such things as an enlarged prostate gland, or prostatitis, an infection in the gland. He sounded reassuring and told me, "This is something we need to follow-up, but it may not be a problem."

———◦•◦◦◦◦◦•◦———

I remembered that I had prostatitis in medical school. Sherry and I had been trying to conceive a child with no luck. She went through a careful evaluation by her gynecologist and was pronounced healthy—no reason why she couldn't get pregnant. It was then my turn to visit a doctor and get checked out. Dutifully I made an appointment with an urologist for infertility studies. (What is it in my fate, which places me repeatedly in the hands of urologists?) The doctor told me that I had a low sperm count. He also found a smoldering infection in my prostate gland. I had no symptoms then, but I obediently took the sulfa drugs he prescribed.

On my next visit he began again to talk about my low sperm count. He wanted to take a biopsy of my testicles! I told him that I wanted to give it some thought. I never went back! Someone taking a piece of my testicle was not my idea of a good time. I wasn't that curious! If we could not conceive a child, we'd damn well adopt one!

I had presumed that the course of sulfa drugs had cured my prostatitis. Perhaps not? The prostatitis was probably back. Sure, that would explain a high PSA! I had heard rumors that riding a bicycle or even having a prostate exam could raise one's PSA. Hell! I had a rectal prostate exam just before I had my blood drawn! Maybe that was the problem. One confidant told me that he heard sex could raise the PSA. Lots of reasons not to worry!

<hr />

A few weeks later I cornered Nick in the hall of the emergency department and asked his advice. He agreed that prostatitis was a possibility and suggested a course of antibiotics. On his recommendation, I took a twenty-one day course of Bactrim. Eventually I got around to rechecking my PSA.

It had risen to 12.4!

As I looked at lab dates, I realized that I had stalled for almost ten weeks while the situation deteriorated. Nick told me that I should consider having a biopsy taken from my prostate gland. I didn't really know how that was done, but I knew that I didn't want to find out. He was beginning to sound like the guy who wanted a piece of my testicles thirty years ago. I asked Nick, "Can't an enlarged prostate gland do this?"

"OK," Nick replied. "A blood test for Free PSA will sort that out for you."

Now this isn't "free" as in free lunch. It means that the PSA is free in the bloodstream—not bound to one of a variety of protein carriers. As a rule, only healthy cells produce free PSA. Cancer cells don't. Consequently, if most of the PSA was free, maybe this was not a malignant process.

⚫⚫⚫⚫⚫⚫⚫

I was in the hospital lab the next morning to get a Free PSA. They don't routinely test for Free PSA at my hospital lab, and sent my blood to a down town lab. The results came back in two days. My Free PSA was 4%—not a good number!

As I read the lab sheet it explained: "Data suggests that prostate cancer is associated with a low percentage of Free PSA." I was supposed to have over 25% Free PSA!

Bottom line: This was not an enlarged prostate gland;

it was probably cancer!

That wasn't the only bad news! I noticed that the downtown lab also tested for my total PSA to determine what percentage was "free." They found a PSA value of 15! Our lab had reported only 12.4. I felt a panic rising in my gut. I reminded myself that numbers will vary between labs, but that didn't help much. There was no denying that these numbers were deteriorating. This time I didn't wait until I found Nick around the hospital. I paged him. When I told him the news over the phone, he came down to the Emergency Department.

Up to this point Nick had handled my problem with a casual air. I suspect he was trying not to alarm me. Now, he was all business.

"Mike you need a biopsy."

"I need time to think this over."—An obvious stall. Hell! It worked thirty years ago with another urologist!

"Good," he replied. "You've got two weeks. I'm going to Greece on vacation."

A two week stay of execution! What a relief!

"OK," I said. "I'll let you know then."

In retrospect, it seems amazing that I was willing to dawdle while a cancer grew in my loins—not very rational. However, I have come to realize that we are not very rational creatures when faced with serious illness. I have seen patients and their families ignore "gawdawful" symptoms pretending nothing was amiss. I remember a man with lung cancer coughing up blood for six months,

that he had a smoker's cough. I have seen a
with a huge breast cancer distorting her breast,
adamant that it was just a mole.

Physicians by no means are immune to denial and
irrational behavior. I maintain that we are the worst. I
recall one colleague who developed every symptom of an
acute heart attack: crushing chest pain radiating down the
left arm, nausea, sweats—the works. Convinced that a
heart attack couldn't be happening to him, he went for a
five-mile run to prove his point! God only knows how he
survived that self-abuse before he relented and drove himself to the hospital.

I am beginning to understand how such things can
happen. Any organism will attempt to restrain forces that
threaten its destruction. We can create the dangerous illusion that an illness holds no power over our
lives, when we refuse to recognize that illness. I knew that I was stalling and in denial.
I also knew that I needed time to mentally
prepare myself, not only for the biopsy, but
for the probability that I had cancer.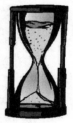

I often urge my patients to take control of their medical care. I believe a physician best serves his patient as a
guide or coach, not as a director. But there's a problem: A
large segment of people don't want to deal with their own
serious illnesses. It's another form of escape. They want
simplistic answers. They want their physician to make the
decisions.

Such behavior always perplexed me! Now I was

beginning to understand these people. I didn't w
deal with this cancer either. I wanted to find the right hit
man to make it go away. I needed a hired gun to chase the
rustlers out of Dodge City.

However, the truth remains. We are ultimately responsible for our care. That's where the buck stops. Accepting
that responsibility brings empowerment. A man
embracing that responsibility can actively participate in
his cure. A take charge attitude provides a sense of mas-
tery over illness. That attitude enables a man to master his
fear. The posse that runs the rustlers out of Dodge begins
to comprehend its power.

Now I was the patient. I needed to embrace my illness. I needed to start making the decisions. It would take
time to educate myself. I knew prostate cancer had a rep-
utation as "Champion Slow Grower." If I had cancer, it
had been there for years. Even though friends beseeched
me to get this settled, I was determined to avoid a precip-
itous decision. Two weeks would be a good start in my
education.

the sometimes empowerment'm
now asks physicians what last

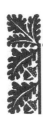

CHAPTER 4

WHAT'S A NICE GUY LIKE YOU
DOING IN STIRRUPS?

I was off duty the next day and headed back to the medical library. I wanted to know what a prostate biopsy really involved. I rummaged through urology textbooks and journals, and once again found the "You Are Here" pictures. There he was again: the eternally suffering patient, lying on his back with his knees up and legs spread—his genitals and rectum exposed. Any woman having a Pap smear knows this position with its inherent vulnerability and discomposure. The surgeon was inserting an ultrasound probe into his rectum to guide the biopsy needle. The biopsy needle was then inserted through the rectum as well.

The rectum has a nerve supply, but not one that notices needle pricks. This means that the procedure is supposed to be relatively painless. The surgeon then routinely takes six specimens through the needle—taking representative samples of the entire gland. The specimens are then sent to the lab for analysis. The rectum is nobody's idea of a sterile place to be sticking needles, and there is a risk of infection. The article recommended antibiotics after the biopsy.

Nick had mentioned the lab's analysis of the biopsy specimen. He said that if cancer were found it would be given a **Gleason Score** from one to ten. High numbers were bad, low numbers not quite so bad. More research to do! Now I had to brush up on the significance of Gleason Scoring.

I was beginning to feel like an over-the-hill doctor! I was encountering concepts that were only developing when I left medical school 27 years ago. Dr. Gleason had not yet published his groundbreaking work. Ultrasound was then in its infancy. Certainly no one was doing ultrasound guided prostate biopsies. This was all well outside my scope of emergency medicine, and I had been only peripherally aware of what was going on.

I remember encountering cancer as a medical student. Cancer had always been a mystery to me. Even the thought of cancer made me uncomfortable then—still does—but I was curious. Just what is it? Why does it happen? What does it do to injure the body that spawns it?

I will never forget my first glimpse of cancer through a microscope. I was studying a slide of lung cancer. What I saw was obviously abnormal tissue. The normal microscopic anatomy was deranged. No longer did I see orderly rows of cells forming the bronchi and air sacks that I had learned to expect. Instead I saw bizarre looking cells with irregular shapes. The nuclei were too big, and the cell contents were stained unevenly. Sometimes the microscopic architecture of the lung was completely destroyed, with nothing but sheets of the bizarre cells filling the microscope. It was apparent that something had gone seriously wrong. Chaos had replaced order. This was anarchy on a cellular level. What had happened to Law and Order?

Normally the human body is a paragon of Law and Order, billions of cells living and working together in harmony. These cells share an amazing wisdom in controlling growth and development. When you grew your left arm, your body knew 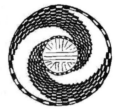 exactly how many fingers to produce, and when to stop growing. Cancer cells won't stop growing. They are intent upon reproducing at all cost. It truly is cellular anarchy. It's every man for himself. The cancer will commandeer the body's resources in competition with normal tissues— the cancer cells eventually crowding out the normal cells. It becomes a parasitic relationship that eventually destroys the host.

———————

Lee Sturgeon-Day has a more poetic definition of cancer:

> In cancer, cells have emancipated themselves from the form and functioning of the body as a whole, and do their own thing at the expense of the total organism. These cells are actually weak and confused, as well they might be, having fallen out of the body's community. Their claim to fame is their capacity to multiply at great speed, sapping the vitality of the body, often to the point of death. We all carry cancer cells, but a healthy organism deals with them effectively. It is only in the cancer patient that the body—or indeed whatever shapes and

guides the body—is unable to destroy them.

A pathologist peering through his microscope can predict which cancers will be bad actors. Basically, the more bizarre the cells look (perhaps confused?), the more malignant the cancer.

Dr. Gleason, a pathologist, did this with prostate cancer in 1978. He studied cancers found in biopsy specimens, and ranked the cancers into five grades. Grade one was the least malignant, grade five the most malignant. Rather than base his opinion on only one specimen, he decided to grade the two worst offenders and add the numbers to produce the **Gleason Score**. For example, if one specimen was graded four, and the next two, he would add them to produce a Gleason Score of six. The lowest possible score now becomes two, the highest ten. And you're right if you're thinking that this could confuse patients. We now have a **Gleason Grade** vs. **Gleason Score**, sometimes called the **Sum**, assigning different numbers to the same cancer.

Subsequent studies inferred that a Gleason Score of ten is grim news. The majority of men with a Gleason Score of ten die of their prostate cancers, regardless of what their doctors do. I found an article in *The New England Journal of Medicine* that correlated mortality and Gleason Scores. In ten years, 66% of those men unlucky enough to have Gleason Scores of 8 to 10 had died. That compares to 13% mortality for those with scores of 7 or less. A score of 2 or 3 is good news. These patients seem to do well in spite of their doctors.

The Gleason Score promised to be a wonderful tool. However, there seem to be two limitations:

❶ Most cancers fall into the intermediate levels of five to seven, where predictions become more vague.

❷ Grading the biopsy specimen is difficult and somewhat subjective. One pathologist may be more impressed with the slides than another pathologist. He may then assign a higher score to a biopsy specimen than the second pathologist might.

Despite those limitations, the Gleason Score is a valuable prognostic tool. It plays a worthwhile role in selecting appropriate therapy.

Any man diagnosed with prostate cancer soon learns this new lexicon, including the terms PSA and Gleason Score. I guarantee you that virtually every man with prostate cancer knows both of his numbers.

As I read all of this, I was feeling detached. The numbers were blurring together, and I didn't really care. Somehow, this didn't seem to apply to me. I expected good news on a biopsy, if I agreed to have one done.

I spent my two-week reprieve struggling with the question of doing a biopsy. Nick had reassured me that if I agreed to a biopsy, he would give me intravenous sedation. I would not remember much about the procedure. I received IV sedation once as a young man, when I had four wisdom teeth pulled. That wasn't so bad. I began to relax. This looked like something I could get through with some grace.

One morning I was lying in bed in that dreamy state between sleep and wakefulness. It had been a restless night filled with images of prostate biopsies. I realized that I was more fearful of the procedure than I was of the possible cancer. I rose from my restless bed and walked into the kitchen to join Sherry for coffee. I had to get this thing behind me. As I sat at the table sipping my brew, I knew that my fears had me paralyzed. That was when I noticed Jeffrey's Nike banner stuck on the refrigerator: "Just Do It!" How simple that made it all seem! Just do it! Of course! Let's get this thing over with, and get back to my life. I called Nick's office and made my appointment for the biopsy.

———◄•••••••►———

The morning of my biopsy, Sherry drove me to Nick's office. I told her I was going to be sedated and would need a ride home. That of course was all male bravado. She knew it. I knew it; and she allowed me to pretend that neither of us knew it. I knew that too. Amazing, the levels of communication that can develop between two people in thirty-five years! I'm aware of the philosophy that we all must face our karma alone, but the truth was: I needed Sherry there. Even though I kept telling myself that this would be no worse than having my wisdom teeth pulled, I was having trouble believing it.

I was out of bed early that morning. I had been a good patient, fasting through the night, and giving myself a morning enema as ordered. I took a long shower afterwards. At least I would be clean if I was going to be exposed on the table.

As I was showering, I recalled a classic story of the battle between the Greeks and Persians at the Pass of Thermopylae. It has always been one of my favorite tales. In 480 B.C., the Persian Army lead by Xerxes had half the known world under its heel and now threatened to overrun Greece. Athens and Sparta refused to surrender, and chose to make their stand at the "Hot Gates" of Thermopylae. There the road ran along the coast, and was sandwiched between the mountains, hot springs, and sea. It narrowed to about fifty feet, and could be easily defended. The Greeks, numbering 7000 strong, were commanded by Leonidas and were vastly outnumbered, perhaps twenty-five to one.

Xerxes received scouting reports that the Greeks were bathing and preening on the eve of the battle. His generals found that quite humorous—until Greek turncoats informed Xerxes that these men were preparing to die.

The Greeks held off Xerxes' human wave for two days, until they were betrayed by their own countrymen. Realizing that the battle was lost, Leonidas addressed his troops at breakfast the third day: "Have a good breakfast men; for tonight we dine in Hades."

I had no intention of dining in Hades anytime soon, but I suspected that this would not be my last ritualistic bath.

⊲●●●●●●●▷

When I arrived at Nick's office, I was warmly greeted

by the staff and promptly ushered into the treatment room by a young nurse, Becky. It was a small room furnished only with an operating table. One wall was covered with shelves of patients' files. Nick's practice appeared to be outgrowing his office space. Becky asked me to disrobe from the waist down and announced that she would be back to give me two antibiotic shots.

Shots? Two? Of course! The antibiotics to prevent infection. Here were two needles I had not anticipated. I suddenly felt a bit unbalanced. I have a theory that each one of us harbors a permanent five-year-old in our psyche. That child is guaranteed to go nuts when anyone approaches with a needle, much less two! My five-year-old was beginning to stir.

As I undressed, I noticed the ultrasound machine. This one looked like a cousin of the Star Wars robot, R2D2, with his finger stuck in his ear. In a show of bravado I pulled R2D2's finger out of his ear. It was the probe designed to fit into my rectum. As Becky returned, I realized the probe was covered with a condom.

"How eminently practical," I commented as I replaced R2D2's finger in his ear.

I climbed onto the treatment table and saw a scary needle set out behind the ultrasound machine. I knew it was meant for me.

"Is that the biopsy needle?"

"Yes," she answered. "Would you like to see it?"

She brought over the longest, fattest needle I had ever seen. It was fastened to a metal cylinder looking vaguely like a syringe. The cylinder was spring-loaded and moved a blade at the end of the needle designed to cut a piece of flesh. She fired it once in demonstration—a foreboding thwack echoed off the walls. Then she had to use two hands to pull the plunger and cock it again! My internal five-year-old was going nuts! I wondered why she was previewing that fearful device. Was this a streak of sadism? I decided that she was simply trying to keep the doctor/patient entertained.

I felt panic as my legs were placed in the stirrups. I struggled with an impulse to abruptly cancel the whole thing, and get the hell out of there! Somewhere I found my resolve to see this through. I considered asking for sedation just as Nick walked in.

"Hi ya Nick. I'da been here earlier, but I couldn't find a thing to wear."

Nick grinned, "Hey, you never looked better."

The scene struck me as socially bizarre. There I was with my crotch exposed to the world, and we were exchanging pleasantries.

"You know, Nick, this would be a good time for the Valium you promised!"

"OK, I got the hint." He reached for the Valium.

Becky reassured me with a comforting smile, "You'll be in LaLa Land in a few minutes and won't remember a thing."

She was right. As Nick injected the medicine, I felt one hell of a drunk coming on.

My next memory was of that spring-loaded contrivance going off somewhere in the core of my body. I had awakened as Nick took the last of six specimens. I truly had felt no pain. Reassured, I drifted off once again into the arms of Morpheus.

I remember awakening again as Nick passed a catheter tube up my penis to my bladder. He was checking for blood. Now that was uncomfortable!

Nick told me, "I examined you while you were asleep. The right lobe of your prostate is more firm than the left. That could be the cancer. I concentrated the biopsy specimens there."

Suddenly one thought pierced through my drunken confusion:

"He expected to find cancer!"

Nick told me that the biopsy went well, and I should have no problems. He then cheerfully announced that there was no blood in my bladder and removed the catheter. Suddenly I was consumed by an overwhelming urge to urinate.

I announced to anyone who would listen, "I need to pee!"

Becky reassured me, "The doctor has just drained your bladder with a catheter. You couldn't possibly need to urinate!"

"Becky, I can't help it! I have to pee!"

"OK, I'll give you a urinal."

With a practiced hand, she unceremoniously slipped my penis into the mouth of a male urinal and left it lying between my legs. And there I lie—like so many old geezers I'd seen before—with my penis in a bottle trying to pee! It had finally come to this.

I was feeling an increasing pain in the head of my penis and couldn't seem to pass any urine. I eventually felt something ooze out of my penis and lifted my head to see what was going on. I was shocked to see blood dripping from the end of my penis! Somehow I was not prepared for that. Everyone else in the room seemed unconcerned. They put my legs down from the stirrups, and gave me time to recover from the sedation. Nick checked on me one more time before I left. He reminded me that the biopsy results would be back in a week. When I was coherent and walking, Sherry took me home.

I will never forget our drive home. I was terribly uncomfortable. I knew that men have difficulty localizing prostate pain. They can't seem to decide where they hurt. I had seen it many times in my practice of medicine. It's called projected pain, and has to do with the way we're wired. Now it was my turn. I was feeling pain at the end of my penis, in my low back, my testicles, my rectum, my right hip—pain projected everywhere except my pelvis. When we arrived home, Sherry gave me pain pills and tucked me into bed. I was eager to find relief in sleep. My curiosity about projected pain had been satisfied.

For the next few days urination was uncomfortable, bloody, and frequent. I had to drink copious fluids to avoid plugging my plumbing with blood clots.

I was startled to see bloody semen. That gradually turned rusty and cleared within two weeks.

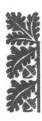

CHAPTER 5

A STITCH IN TIME DOES NOT SAVE MINE.

It was time to visit Nick and discuss my biopsy results. Sherry came with me for the discussion. Once again I needed her support, and she needed to be involved. I was recovered from the biopsy and feeling no symptoms. As we drove to Nick's office, I felt the tension mount. I knew the real agenda was scheduling a prostatectomy. Somehow there had to be an option other than going under the knife.

For me surgery had always seemed a brutal affair. In medical school I had endured an aggressive, egotistical surgery professor who delighted in declaring, "The whole world is pre-op." My standard reply became, "If the Good Lord intended for us to have surgery, he would have designed in a zipper." I have indelible memories of my surgical rotation as a medical student. I remember my back aching as I retracted a patient's liver—while an attending physician rummaged in the patient's abdomen.

One of my most vivid memories is the first amputation I helped perform. I had just finished my first year of medical school, and was doing summer study with a renowned orthopaedic surgeon. Our mission was to remove the gangrenous leg of an unfortunate diabetic patient. I was holding the man's leg with my left hand, while the orthopaedist sawed through the femur. I had an artery clamp in my other hand. My job was to clamp the femoral artery if the bleeding became severe. Suddenly the leg was free. I was surprised by its weight and almost dropped the leg onto the floor. *GROSSED OUT!* I handed the amputated leg to a waiting nurse. I'll long remember the blood draining onto the floor as she took it away.

It was days before I could go back into the surgery suite. Even today I get a creepy feeling as I pass the doors to the Surgery Department. I couldn't imagine entering those doors on a stretcher.

<hr>

I was busy after my biopsy. A colleague recommended a book by Michael Korda: *Man to Man, Surviving Prostate Cancer.* I devoured the book in three days. It was a Godsend. Mr. Korda tells the story of his prostate cancer in sensitive, honest dialogue. He is older than I. His Gleason Score and PSA values were similar. He chose a radical prostatectomy for his therapy and traveled to Johns Hopkins University Medical Center for surgery by Dr. Patrick C. Walsh, director of the Department of Urology and a world class surgeon. He has developed a surgical technique for prostatectomy—sparing the nerves controlling a man's erection and reducing his risk of impotence.

Mr. Korda described trials as he moved towards surgery. I was comforted by his admissions of doubts and fears, many of which I was feeling. I was troubled by his graphic descriptions of surgery and recovery. He had a turbulent post-operative course, plagued by urine incontinence. At one point he was sleeping between rubber sheets. As the book ended, he was nine months post-surgery and on the road to recovery. He was still impotent. I didn't want to follow in his footsteps.

We arrived at Nick's office at 5 PM. He had scheduled my visit at the end of his day so that we could talk undisturbed. Again we were greeted warmly by his staff who informed us: "The Doctor is tied up in surgery and will not be available for about an hour." His secretary gave us the option of rescheduling the appointment. There was no way I could postpone this conversation any longer. We agreed to wait for Nick.

That was one of the longest hours of my life! I felt panic rising as I sat in the waiting room. I became restless, paced the floor, wandered outside, tried to read—all to no avail. I felt oppression building in my chest. I suddenly needed fresh air again. I reminded myself that Nick could not operate on me unless I agreed. That helped a bit. Sherry was doing a better job of containing herself, but I could see the tension in her posture.

On the reading table I found a booklet describing prostate cancer. It explained the four stages of the cancer. I knew that if I could focus on the facts, it would take my mind off my panic. Besides, I would need to review that information to talk intelligently with Nick. My treatment would be based on the stage of my cancer. "**Staging**" a patient's cancer is critical to his care.

The booklet explained a staging system using the letters A, B, C, and D. Stage D is the worst. Stage D implies that the cancer has **metastasized**—spread to distant tissues and set up housekeeping. Stage A is the least treacherous—notice I didn't say best—and assumes that the cancer is confined to the prostate gland. A physician cannot feel this cancer on rectal prostate exam. Stage B cancers are palpable, but otherwise cause no symptoms. Stage C cancers are rock hard on digital rectal examination, because the cancer has usually occupied all of the prostate. Typically these cancers extend through the capsule, invading surrounding tissue. Patients bearing stage C malignancies are often diagnosed after they have developed symptoms, most commonly trouble urinating.

I was aware that there is a second staging system out there which assigns numbers T0 through T4 (T for "Tumor"), with subcategories a, b, and c, and further designations for positive lymph nodes and metastases. This system is used in academic circles, but seems unwieldy for many men with prostate cancer.

Reading the pamphlet didn't help. I was still restless. I walked out to the car and turned on the stereo. I laid the seat back and closed my eyes—didn't help either. I found a journal article I had tossed onto the back seat. A concerned partner had given it to me. It was a "throw-away journal" about prostate cancer. The headline sounded encouraging: "Survival Is High Ten Years After Prostatectomy." Excellent! I could use some good news right now.

Hungrily I pounced on the article. It came from the University of Chicago Pritzker School of Medicine. The authors told a tale of 2,758 men diagnosed with early prostate cancer and scheduled for radical prostatectomy. At surgery the surgeons discovered that 91 of those men had been staged wrong! They did not have early cancer. The surgeons found the cancer in neighboring lymph nodes and canceled the surgery. The surgeons just closed the incisions and sent these men to the recovery room. They were excluded from the study.

The remaining 2,667 men underwent a radical prostatectomy. Eighty-five percent were still living 10 years later. Seventy percent had no evidence of disease. The authors were evidently pleased with those numbers.

I didn't share their exuberance at all! A survival rate of 85% meant that 400 men had died. A cure rate of 70% meant that 800 men still had cancer 10 years after surgery.

There was also the group of 91 unfortunate men who went to surgery, had their abdomens opened, and then closed. They awoke in the recovery room to the news that their cancer was beyond surgery. I tried to imagine how that must feel. My brain simply wouldn't do it. It went into tilt instead. I just sat there dumbfounded, until I noticed Nick's Mercedes pulling into the parking lot. I waved a greeting and went back to the waiting room in a state of agitated depression.

Sherry was alone in the room. Most of Nick's staff had gone home. Nick appeared a few minutes later. He had slipped in a private door. Still wearing his surgical greens, he looked weary after a day of surgery. He invited us into his office. On my way into the room, I noticed pictures of his family in Greece. One lovely elderly lady had to be his mother. I relaxed a bit when I saw Nick's desk piled with paperwork and unread journals. I muttered, "A neat desk is a sign of a sick mind," and smiled to myself. Nick settled back in his leather chair with his feet up, obviously enjoying a chance to sit down and relax a bit. Me? I was too nervous to sit. I stood there as we spent some time exchanging pleasantries.

Then Nick turned serious.

"Mike, I'm sorry I had to give you that news over the phone. It must have felt like a sledge hammer. I'm glad we finally have a chance to talk. I have the final results of your biopsy. That phone call was just a preliminary report. Your biopsy has been given a Gleason Score of six."

Damn! A Gleason Score of Six! I had been hoping for better news. Even though I knew the majority of Gleason scores were five to seven, I was hoping for a two or three. I began to feel the situation deteriorating. Suddenly, I was moving through a Shakespearian tragedy. I found myself thinking of Macbeth. He begins his story confident of his success. He was buoyed on the promises by dark spirits that "no man born of woman" could harm him. However, as the plot unfolds we see him blindly moving towards his

52

eventual doom despite his optimism. I did not want to be doomed to a painful death of metastatic prostate cancer.

Nick told me that I had many options to consider, and that I had time to think about what I wanted to do.

"Mike, I think I can cure you. I recommend a prostatectomy." I noticed that he left off the word *radical* when he spoke of surgery—good work.

"What kind of recovery are we talking about Nick?"

"The surgery of course is done under anesthesia. After that you'll be in the hospital about five days. You won't feel much pain. I'll do an epidural morphine drip for you."

I explained to Sherry that for "an epidural" a small catheter is placed next to the spinal nerves of the lower back, the epidural space. Morphine is dripped into the space as needed to control pain. Pretty high tech pain control—works well. I found that reassuring.

Nick went on. "You'll be home recovering for a month or two, maybe three."

"How come so long?" I asked.

"Well, you'll have a catheter in your bladder for two to six weeks for one thing, and you may have some temporary urine incontinence."

For the first time I began to appreciate what a financial impact this could have on my family. Three months of lost income would certainly threaten my financial house of cards. I've seen this happen to my patients. Telling a man that he is having a heart attack, for example, produces great financial echoes. How many of us could tolerate three months of lost income? Failing health is the most common cause of bankruptcy. I forced down the financial alarm and attempted to focus on the conversation.

I mentioned that I had read about Dr. Walsh and his nerve sparing operation. I asked Nick if he used that procedure.

"Yes, of course!" he replied.

I decided to ask the hard question as tactfully as possible.

"Nick, do you feel deep in your heart that you are the best man to do my surgery?"

Did I hear defiance in my voice? To be perfectly honest, I wasn't feeling very tactful. I was feeling cornered and increasingly angry.

Nick was taken aback a bit. He paused to think and finally said:

"Michael, if I were you, I would find the very best super-surgeon I could find for my prostatectomy. That way if things did not go well, at least I would be able to say that I gave it my best shot."

I was disappointed with that answer. I had expected Nick to stand up for himself. However, I realized that ours was not a pure doctor-patient relationship. We were also colleagues. I agree that I could be a threatening patient— with possibly unrealistic expectations. I suspected that Nick simply did not want to complicate his life or our relationship. He probably was intuitively aware of my rising anger, at least on some level. No physician wants his competence questioned at every turn, nor would he want responsibility for a colleague's care if things go badly. Caring for one's friends or family can be difficult, especially if complications arise.

I remembered Michael Korda's book. He had gone to Baltimore for his surgery. He felt so devastated after the surgery that he abandoned his plans to fly home to New York on a commercial aircraft. He actually chartered a medical transport aircraft to take him home. An ambulance met him at the airport. I didn't have that caliber of financial resources. The thought of going out of town for the care of a superstar surgeon seemed fraught with logistical difficulties. I couldn't imagine getting on an airplane—with a catheter protruding from my penis—five days after a prostatectomy.

I also had a heart connection to Nick. I knew that if he were given the opportunity, he would provide me with the very best care he could. That was crucial to me. If I were to have surgery, I wanted it to be in my hospital, surrounded by my people—people I had come to know over the past twenty years.

I quietly decided that Nick would be my man—IF I decided to have surgery.

As the conversation began to wind down, Nick asked if we had any questions. Sherry surprised me with a question for Nick.

"Nick, what would you do if this were you?"

Nick smiled, leaned back in his chair and said: "Sherry, I'll tell you a little secret. I have never had my PSA tested. I don't want to have to deal with this myself.

I have no idea what I would do. If I decided not to have surgery, I would consider going to Seattle to have radioactive seeds implanted into my prostate gland."

Now that was interesting! I had never heard of radioactive seeds used in such a way.

Realizing that Sherry and I were coming on strong, I tried to lighten up the conversation. I announced: "Yeah, Nick's a lot older than I am. He doesn't have to worry about long term effects."

Nick smiled and countered, "Not that much older. I think you should give yourself time to think about all the options. We could put you on hormone suppression therapy for a while. You might not have to do anything for years. We will have plenty of time to talk again and decide what you want to do."

I felt adrift. Although I was impressed with the way that Nick left me in control, I had actually expected more direction. Nick's agenda that evening appeared limited. He intended to review my biopsy report, and begin a discussion of my options. He probably considered it obvious that I should have a prostatectomy. He wasn't going to tell me what to do. He invited us to return for more conversation—after I had an opportunity to think a bit.

I realized that we were now alone with Nick in the building. His staff had quietly departed, and Nick was looking tired. The day was darkening, and I had plenty to think about. Time to go. We excused ourselves, shook hands, and made a loose commitment to get together for more conversation.

Sherry and I spoke only briefly on the drive home. I was lost in my own thoughts. I was struck with the stark reality of my situation: "Damn! I really do have cancer! *What am I going to do?*" I had to start making a decision! It wouldn't be the last time I wrestled with that question.

And then there's the great irony: "I have just been counseled by a physician who has never tested his own PSA!" I didn't see this as especially illogical—rather as a confession of futility. No one is sure that all this effort is doing much good! Besides, who ever said that physicians are any more rational than the rest of us?

I pondered how many men have been rendered impotent, sterile, or incontinent in the name of therapy—for a disease that seemed to take its own indolent course over ten years. How many men could have gone to their graves happy and unaware that they had prostate cancer—if they never tested their PSA? Instead they risked death in surgery, or bloody bowel movements from their radiation therapy, simply because a blood test has been developed.

Nick had told me that about a third of prostate cancer patients do well without any therapy, a third do poorly 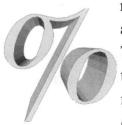 regardless of therapy, and about a third actually benefit from their doctors' care. That means that two thirds don't need all the expense and heroics. Problem is that no one knows how to find the third that do!

In Nick's defense, I knew that the National Cancer Institute maintains *there is no evidence that PSA testing or rectal prostate exams decrease mortality*. Meanwhile the American Cancer Society and American Urological Association insist that rectal prostate exams and PSA testing should begin at age fifty. I knew that entire countries, such as Great Britain and Canada, believe such testing produces more mischief than good. They don't recommend routine PSA testing. I began to suspect that Nick was showing some wisdom in his decision to avoid PSA testing.

Despite this confusion, the California State Legislature couldn't resist getting involved. It seems that the politicians are increasingly willing to tell physicians how to practice good medicine, even when no one is sure what "good medicine" really is. So now the government is looking over my shoulder every time I do a rectal exam. As of 1997, every time I examine a patient's prostate gland, I must counsel him about available PSA testing "if the patient is over fifty, manifests clinical symptoms, is at increased risk for prostate cancer, or the provision of the information is medically necessary." This is now mandated by law! It's just a matter of time before some poor physician gets snared in a hopeless malpractice suit by this one.

I have a colleague who insists, "Much of the rest of the world is less surgically inclined than we Americans. They look in bemusement at our cowboy heroics."

I hoped to avoid heroics. One could possibly contain this illness without heroics and live with it, much as patients live with other chronic illnesses such as Diabetes

Mellitus or high blood pressure. I began to see that the real purpose of my therapy would be dying of something else.

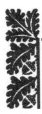

CHAPTER 6

BABY BUGGIES EVERYWHERE!

My secret was out. I began to talk freely to friends at work. This cancer was beginning to consume my life, if not my body. There was no way I could keep such news from my co-workers. We were simply too close—a closeness born of eighteen years together in the human struggle against disease.

I was especially impressed by Pattie, our department secretary. She has survived breast cancer. She has endured a mastectomy, chemotherapy, and breast reconstruction. She has been bald and has worn wigs—the whole shebang. Looking at this self-confident woman now, one would never suspect what she has been through. She now sports a full head of lovely hair, which compliments a shapely figure. She is actively involved in supporting other women with breast cancer.

She approached me with a big hug and encouragement.

"I heard the news, Doctor. You know you are going to survive this. If I did it, you can." She smiled, "You *will* laugh again." She told me that I was going through the most difficult period for a cancer patient. "The reality that you have cancer confronts you. It's scary that the decisions you make now are so irreversible! You will need to live with them for the rest of your life. What is most scary will appear during those times when you are alone with your thoughts. You will realize that this is real and that people die with cancer!"

She put her hands on my shoulders and looked me in the eyes. "I know that this will sound strange, and you will probably tell me that I'm nuts. I'll say it anyway. I would never have asked for my cancer or what I went through, but I would never give it up now. You are going to experience one of the most dynamic periods of your life. It will change you forever."

Her final advice was: "This thing will consume you for a while. That's OK. Read everything you can get your hands on. Talk to as many people as you can. Give them a chance to support you. You will find that they really do want to contribute to you. Don't worry about becoming a bore. Give yourself into this process; you need to work through it."

Later that day I found myself having coffee with a couple of other physicians. One greeted me with, "Hey Mike, howyadoin?" I decided to take Pattie's advice and *really* share how I was "doin'." I smiled slightly and simply said "I have cancer!" My announcement fell into the conversation like a hand grenade. I began to sense the power such news held. My embarrassment was falling away. I actually began to enjoy my power to usurp the center of attention anytime I chose. I would need to be careful lest I become a bore—Let's talk about me and my prostate cancer!

I confided that I was still struggling with a plan of action. One doc told me, "I've recently heard of a new technique to kill the cancer by freezing the prostate gland. You might want to look into that." One physician, a retired surgeon, had performed surgery with Nick many times. I asked his opinion of Nick's skills.

"Nick really knows his way around in the pelvis. He's a fine technician—has good hands." The phrases "fine technician" and "good hands" are about as good as it gets. That's ultimate praise from another surgeon. I was encouraged. I renewed my decision to stay with Nick.

A third Doc, also a surgeon, advised me: "Set aside some blood of your own before the surgery—at least two units. That surgery gets pretty bloody! You'll need the blood." My mouth felt dry as I thanked him for that advice.

I began to see the wisdom in Pattie's counsel. These men really did want to contribute to the waves of support I knew I would need to come through this. I just had to give them the chance.

I knew it was time to get serious about researching the literature. I needed to learn everything about prostate cancer *fast*! I called the medical library and told the librarian my story. She was so confident and professional, that speaking to her was a delight. She reassured me: "I have heard this story from several doctors lately. I've become an expert on doing literature searches on prostate cancer. I'll have a bibliography ready for you in the morning."

There it was again, a hint that something unusual was happening in the world of prostate cancer. The librarian had developed expertise in finding information for doctors—doctors with their own prostate cancers!

I remember the first time I became a father. We adopted Tammy—age four days. This perfect baby girl just had to have the perfect baby buggy. Sherry and I spent three days picking out that perfect buggy. Suddenly I was noticing baby buggies everywhere. The world was full of people pushing baby buggies. How could I have been so blind to them?

Now prostate cancer seemed to be everywhere! Had I discovered a tidal shift in this disease, or was this just another baby buggy phenomenon?

That evening I resolved to "Surf the Net" and see what I could find on the World Wide Web. Sitting at my computer, I found a search program and typed in the words: 'Prostate Cancer' and 'Gleason Score.' The program found over ninety-six thousand references! I was flabbergasted. I was profoundly impressed with what 'World Wide' really meant. I had tapped into the world's sum total of knowledge. I was beginning to comprehend the enormity of the task before me. I couldn't follow up on ninety-six thousand references in a lifetime. How was I going to make sense of all of this? I understood how a patient could just capitulate, just put himself in the hands of the first physician he encountered.

I started to sample the references. I found one web site entitled *My Story* where men are invited to tell their stories of prostate cancer. These men are willing to share the intimate details of their illnesses with the world. I made a mental note that I might one day submit my story. I found chat rooms for families as well as patients. Support groups provided inspirational verses, stories of successes, advice, and even more references. I learned that many universities and medical centers supported web sites about prostate cancer. Most were extolling the virtues of their facilities and staff, but they provided a wealth of basic information as well.

I found innumerable books about prostate cancer on the net. A few phone calls and a credit card can produce more than anyone could read. I read excerpts from a powerful book—*Affirming the Darkness*—by Chuck and Martha Wheeler. They kept journals as they battled Chuck's prostate cancer over eight years. Chuck ultimately succumbed to his cancer. Martha finished the book. This deeply moving story illustrates how prostate cancer profoundly affects both a man *and his wife.* I recommend it.

I even stumbled across a web site maintained by Theragenics Corporation. This company manufactures the radioactive seeds mentioned by Nick—good information.

I began frantically printing items as I found them on the Net. I was so immersed and driven that I lost all track of time. By 3:00 AM I had exhausted our supply of computer paper. I sat there at my desk, likewise exhausted, staring at my work. Was there time to digest all of this or was I just kidding myself? Was I stalling, wasting time, while this beast flourished in my groin? Was sleep deprivation weakening my ability to resist this beast?

My thoughts turned to Sherry. She had gone to bed alone five hours earlier. There would be no lovemaking tonight. I had just spent hours reading men's tales of their lost sexuality. How much time did Sherry and I have left as lovers? What an idiot I was, to let her go to bed alone! I had an irrational urge to rush into the bedroom, awaken my lady, sweep her into my arms in passionate embrace, and spend the night in love. Such a beautiful woman and so little time! The song *Just Give Me One More Night* raced through my mind. Somewhere between fear and fatigue my determined research degenerated to cliches and song lyrics.

Enough! I switched off the computer and went into the bedroom. I undressed in the darkness to avoid disturbing Sherry. I could hear her rhythmic breathing as she slept. I was thankful for her steadfast love. I knew that she would stand by me no matter what our common destiny. Was I destined to become an old man smelling vaguely of urine, dribbling pee every time I coughed? I'd seen such men many times on hospital rounds. How could Sherry find me attractive wearing adult diapers?

It was at that moment, standing next to my sleeping bride of thirty-three years, that I made a critical resolution: Whatever therapy I chose, I would be willing to accept an increased risk of dying, if I could preserve my sexuality. I also vowed to do whatever I could to avoid becoming a urological cripple. That determination would become my compass, as I worked to set a course in—what was for me—the uncharted wilderness of cancer.

I snuggled under the covers close to my lady, feeling a little sorry for myself. I remembered Nick's odds of fifty percent impotence after a radical prostatectomy. Snuggling had always been an important part of our intimate moments. Would that be enough to sustain us if I were to find myself impotent?

I know several men who are using artificial methods to produce an erect penis. The wonders of science are out there waiting to salvage a frustrated sexuality. I have seen men with penile implants producing a permanent erection, of sorts. I imagined the difficulties of trying to wear a bathing suit in public with one of those in place. Now there is a penile implant that is inflatable. Yes inflatable! A surgeon permanently implants two long, sausage-shaped bladders in the shaft of the penis. A small ball pump fits into the scrotum. Squeezing one's scrotum a few times will produce a serviceable erection. One man I know chose to have the inflatable implant. He actually winked at me once and bragged that he could now perform all night, if he chose.

I will never forget one unfortunate man who once

appeared in the Emergency Department during the wee morning hours. He had suffered an automobile accident many years previously and been paralyzed from the waist down. He had lost all nerve supply to his genitals. With no sensation in his penis, he could not get an erection. His physician had taught him how to produce an erection by injecting medicine into the shaft of his penis. Apparently he and his lady had used too much medicine that night. His erection had persisted for six hours and he was alarmed. He knew that he could injure his penis if the erection lasted much longer.

In all honesty, I had not encountered this in thirty years of practicing medicine. I had to phone poor Nick at three AM for advice. He recommended an injectable antidote and told me that I had to massage the penis for about fifteen minutes after the injection. With a bit of trepidation, I injected the medicine into my patient's penis, and spent about fifteen minutes massaging his penis with the help of his lady friend. The whole scene seemed surreal to me. I never thought I'd be so glad to see an erection go away. I was genuinely impressed with the power of modern drugs to produce an erection.

I know a man who has been rendered impotent by a prostatectomy. He injects the same medication into his penis every time he has sexual intercourse. He seems content to do that to preserve his sexual life.

Personally, the thought of sticking a needle down there gives me the shivers—definitely not my idea of foreplay. In my role of a sexually potent Caregiver, these artificial contrivances had always seemed a bit desperate to me. Now, I wasn't so sure. I have never walked in the shoes of these men. I hoped that I never would have to find out how desperate I could become.

The next morning Sherry and I were drinking coffee. I told her about my thoughts last night. I shared my apprehensions about becoming impotent and undesirable. It wasn't easy. Sherry came over to me and held me in her arms.

"Michael, I married you for who you are, not for your penis."

What an incredible woman! In one clear declarative sentence she had washed away my fears. She gave me room to move and breathe. Our marriage could survive this. We could survive this.

One of my most vivid childhood experiences happened at age seven. I was furious at my mother for insisting that I needed a bath. I refused to bathe. As I stomped out of the room, I angrily exclaimed: "I wish I could have a new mommy!"

My grandfather, who had witnessed my outburst, found me outside a few minutes later. He had a Sears catalogue in his hand.

"You know Michael, I think you're right. Time to pick out a new mommy."

I wasn't sure if he was kidding or not. He had a smile on his face as he opened the book. He had found the women's underwear pages. Here was page after page of smiling women in bras and panties, all waiting to be picked as a new mommy. Grandpa began to look serious as he continued.

"First we'll pick out a mommy who will feed us anything we want to eat, and let you get as dirty as you want. Then we'll pick out some new clothes for her in the dress section. I think we can have a new one in about three days."

Whether Grandpa was inspired or just thought he was being funny, I'll never know. He didn't even remember the incident when I mentioned it ten years later, but I'll never forget it. I was suddenly faced with the reality of replacing my mother! As I looked at those photos of women in undergarments, I was aghast. I knew this would not do! No barren, plastic, Sears Roebuck mommy was capable of replacing my mother! At age seven I understood that human relationships are not disposable. My mother and I had inseparable bonds of love that would not be severed by a fantasy mom from Sears!

I was suddenly overcome with embarrassment for my behavior, and a love for my mother. I ran into the house to embrace her and apologize for my behavior. She welcomed me with open arms, confirming our love. I had learned an unforgettable lesson in the school of life, course title: **Committed Relationships 101**.

Speaking of committed relationships, I have a confession to make. I occasionally enjoy checking out the personal ads in our local newspaper. I really believe that most of us read them from time to time. I'm just willing to admit it. I seem to stumble across them every few months as I drink my morning coffee. Seeking romance through a personal advertisement is a whole segment of life I've never experienced. It's been thirty-four years since I was a single man. I'm definitely not in the market, but I enjoy what I've dubbed my Prince Charming Fantasy. I will read the ads and try to pick out the most interesting woman (kind of like the Sears catalogue?). I try to imagine what it would be like to call one of them and become part of her life—to arrive on my white horse and sweep her off her feet, like a modern Prince Charming.

Part of the exercise also involves writing my own advertisement. Now that is a real challenge of late.

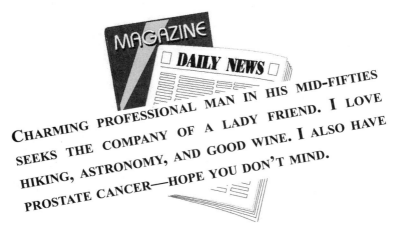

CHARMING PROFESSIONAL MAN IN HIS MID-FIFTIES SEEKS THE COMPANY OF A LADY FRIEND. I LOVE HIKING, ASTRONOMY, AND GOOD WINE. I ALSO HAVE PROSTATE CANCER—HOPE YOU DON'T MIND.

I understood that I was not very marketable. Prince Charming never had to worry about impotence, incontinence, or dying early. Thank God I have a woman who loves me and is willing to stand by me.

I began to appreciate how many positive things I had going for me. I had financial resources at my disposal. I had knowledge of my disease and the ability to find out what I didn't know. I had an immensely supportive circle of friends, both personally and professionally. I had a spiritual concept of life and its trials that gave significance to my illness. I had a loving wife who would be there no matter what.

I often see patients who are so destitute, they have none of the above. It seems miraculous to me that they survive *any* illness. If I couldn't survive this cancer, who could? Comforted by this knowledge, I resolved to beat this thief that threatened to steal the golden years of my life.

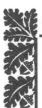

CHAPTER 7

PERHAPS THERE IS NO BEST THERAPY.

Eager to start my search for the right cure, I arrived early at the medical library. The librarian gave me her bibliography of recent articles and I wandered into the stacks to find the journals. These journals all had lighthearted names such as *Cancer*, or *The American Journal of Urology*, or *The International Journal of Radiation Oncology*. As I had anticipated, they were professional, erudite, learned, and damned difficult to read. After thirty years of exposure, I still find it difficult to read medical journals. My eyes glaze over and my mind mutinies. This morning, however, I was a driven man, determined to get to the core of the issues. My task was to review the therapy of early prostate cancer and select the right one for me. I accepted my Herculean task with the vigor of a modern day Grecian hero. I was soon surrounded with journals, tables, computer print outs, and textbooks. By lunchtime I was still in the preliminary stages of my reading. The librarian announced that she was going to lunch and could lock me in the building if I wished. I accepted her offer and pressed on, skipping lunch, and now literally locked in this struggle.

By suppertime I'd had enough. I had

hoped to find answers. What I found was even more questions. I was far from knowing what I had hoped to learn, and my brain was full. I scooped up arms full of material for home review. As I stopped to thank the librarian, she smiled and offered me encouragement:

"Most of the doctors find this tough at first."

How had she sensed my frustration? Was I that transparent, or has she seen this before? She was right. I was frustrated, angry, frightened, and singularly confused.

On my drive home I relaxed and tried to sort through my impressions of a day's reading. I saw a few truths emerging:

⇨ The discovery of PSA about ten years ago has changed the playing field. Because PSA testing provides early detection of prostate cancer, unsuspecting men are receiving the bad news at a younger age. As the patients become younger, their demands for a permanent cure become more strident. They emphasize the concerns of younger men—especially their sexuality.

⇨ Prostate cancer is a slow growing malignancy. Patients must be observed many years before changes in their therapy can be evaluated. There are only a few studies following patients for ten years post-therapy. Even fewer can claim fifteen years. PSA testing has changed that too. It appears that physicians can predict who will survive after therapy by following their PSA levels. Essentially if a patient's PSA remains low for a few years, he's probably cured. Of course, there are physicians vehemently disputing that assumption.

⇨ In fact, consensus was hard to find anywhere! I began to realize that this was one source of my frustration. Cruising home on the freeway, I had one of those rare flashes of clarity! *Perhaps there is no best therapy*! What I *had* found is an ongoing argument raging primarily between the radiologists and the surgeons. Both groups claim to have the *Gold Standard* of therapy. Both camps produce papers comparing their work to the other, often couched in polite condescension.

The urological surgeons state that unless cancer is imprisoned in a bottle, there is no real cure. Some state that a patient refusing surgery risks a relapse in a few years. The radiologists insist that the genie is already out of the bottle about a third of the time, even at early diagnosis. Some imply that a third of new patients have cancer extending through the capsule of their prostate glands on the day they hear they have prostate cancer.

A study out of Johns Hopkins suggests this extracapsular extension of the cancer is a major cause of cancer recurrence. A patient with extracapsular extension has a 60% chance of cancer recurrence after radical prostatectomy. Possibly cancer cells are spilled into the bed of the prostate when it is removed at surgery—at least that's one speculation. A related analysis out of Johns Hopkins has produced the **Partin Tables**, which predict one's odds of having extracapsular extension. These tables represent a tectonic shift in our thinking about prostate cancer. Dr. Partin's team followed a large number of surgical patients for ten years. They examined the prostate glands removed at surgery to see who had cancer invading through the

75

capsule. They then correlated these results to the PSA and Gleason Scores. They added a third factor: the clinical presentation (staging) of the cancer. They then created the **Partin Tables**, using all three numbers.

If a patient knows his PSA, Gleason Score, and clinical stage of cancer, he can look in the Partin Tables and see the risk of capsule penetration for his cancer. In my case, that risk was as high as 73%! And if 60% of the time that penetrating cancer recurs after prostatectomy, my post surgical risk of recurrent cancer was 44%! (Just take 60% of 73%.) Crummy odds!

Incarcerating my cancer in a laboratory bottle would not be easy. No wonder I was so uneasy after a day at the library. I had just calculated that I had only a 56% chance of a surgical cure. There had to be a better answer. I was not willing to accept odds little better than 50/50 after going through the trauma of surgery. Perhaps my cure lay outside the surgical theater.

That evening was a somber one. I found myself imagining what it might be like to die of metastatic prostate cancer. I tried not to dwell on the thought too long, lest I create that reality for myself.

I've enjoyed reading Eastern Philosophy, especially as it applies to illness. One basic tenant is that *thoughts have creative power*. Depak Chopra sums it up by saying: "Nature goes to exactly the same place to create a thought as it goes to create a galaxy." I do believe that Chopra is onto something here. This is more than just magical thinking. I had to maintain a positive attitude.

Another sage who has influenced me is the Austrian philosopher, Rudolf Steiner. He stressed the importance of committing to a decision as soon as possible. It isn't until one is committed that the angels can begin to act.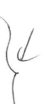

This decision was taking too long. That evening I decided to seriously explore radiation therapy. Meanwhile, tomorrow would be a busy day. Bradley Barnhill had ordered several diagnostic tests to see just how far my cancer had really spread.

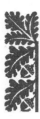

CHAPTER 8

BUT FIRST WE HAVE TO DO A FEW STUDIES.

The next morning I was up early and hit the road. Bradley had planned a busy day for me. We were to complete staging my cancer. The big question of the day: how much has this malignancy spread? A critical question! Inaccurate staging is a major cause of treatment failure. I was determined to avoid that mistake. I would discover as much as humanly possible about the extent of my cancer.

I had the first appointment of the day for Magnetic Resonance Imaging (MRI). The radiologist would be targeting my pelvis. After that I'd receive a chest x-ray and a bone scan. This would be a total body survey, searching those places a cancer might be hiding. I was optimistic. The odds were with me. With a PSA of 10 to 15, there was little chance that we'd find a hidden cancer.

I was also aware that my medical plan would be paying big bucks. These are expensive studies. I'm sure their bean counters considered this a waste of money. I didn't care! I didn't care about saving their money. I didn't care about their probability tables. I needed to know! So much for the rational conservation of medical resources.

Entering the **MRI** suite felt like entering the twenty-fourth century. This is revolutionary technology that reminds me of *Star Trek*. It allows physicians to peer into a body as never before. Even with my degree in physics, I barely understand how this fabulous machine works—just barely.

For my **Magnetic Resonance Imaging**, I would be placed into the core of a super magnet—a magnet using electrical coils super-cooled with liquid helium to minus 450 degrees Fahrenheit. The extremely cold temperature changes the wires' physical properties, making them super-conducting. That's the only way they can handle the incredible electrical currents needed to generate the magnetic field—a magnetic field thousands of times greater than that generated by the Earth itself! The magnetic field would line up atoms in my body's water and fat. These atoms would then be energized with pulses of radio waves. It's somewhat akin to microwave cooking. In fact, I've heard that the patients actually warm up a bit. When the molecules release that energy again, they radiate new radio waves. Antennae around my body would pick up those signals. A powerful computer then turns those signals into an image. Pretty amazing! This machine is housed in a specially shielded room to eliminate outside electromagnetic interference, and to contain those generated by the MRI.

Of course, a patient may not have a MRI if his body contains some types of metal found in artificial heart valves, aneurysm clips, pacemakers, hearing aids, etc. One of my friends advised me to keep my credit cards well away from the machine. The magnetic strips on my cards could be erased. Another recommended that I wear a sweat suit because the tube is cold.

Believe it or not this is listed as a "non-invasive" technology. It's considered safe and painless. It appears safer than using ionizing radiation such as x-rays or bone scans. Nevertheless, I had misgivings about putting my body into a claustrophobic tube surrounded by liquid helium— to be barraged by concentrated radio waves in a formidable magnetic field. Even if this doesn't affect my body, what in heaven does this do to my soul?

The actual experience was not so bad. I emptied my pockets and placed my watch in a locker next door. I left my shoes on for the procedure and climbed onto a narrow stretcher at the mouth of the tube, knowing I was sure to be warm and cozy in my sweat suit. A technician offered me earphones and asked me what radio station I preferred. As he moved the stretcher into the magnet, my feet began to move about and refused to go into the tube. Of course! I had metal shanks in the soles of my Rockports. I had to shed the shoes.

Now barefooted, I entered the tube. I was shocked by how claustrophobic I felt! I seemed to barely fit into the tube. My arms were pinned tightly against my sides. My face seemed no more than three inches from the top of the tube. I was rapidly overcome with claustrophobia and demanded release from the confinement!

I was surprised to see myself become so distraught. I have endured claustrophobic situations in the past with impunity. As a flight surgeon in the USAF, I'd spent many hours in the back seats of high performance aircraft. Now that's claustrophobic! An airman (actually called the "stuffer") would help me strap my fanny to an ejection seat, sitting on top of a cannon shell in a supersonic aircraft. I would be wearing a G-suit designed to squeeze every drop of blood out of my lower extremities on tight turns. I wore a helmet with a face shield, and when I looked up I saw the canopy just a few inches over my head. One aircraft had a short knife attached to the canopy that I could use to cut my way out if necessary. No Problem! The ejection seat was designed to blow right through the canopy if it failed to open. Still, I never felt claustrophobic. I think it's safe to say that I'm not claustrophobic.

The technician offered to reschedule me for another try—under sedation. He also advised me that there was a larger MRI downtown for big patients that seemed less confining. No, I was determined to get this done. The tech tried another approach. He promised to let me out if I panicked—the minute I hollered. That would work! With that feeling of control I knew I could get through the study. Once again I was entombed in the tube. I kept my eyes closed and envisioned myself on the beach.

The MRI itself was a study in sound effects. It sounded as if I had fallen into a giant meat grinder. This meat grinder had a gnome loose somewhere in its bowels that would randomly bang on the pipes with a monkey wrench. This was high tech? In retrospect, the most daunting part of the test was lying perfectly still for half an hour.

————◄•••••••••————

When I was freed, the radiologist invited me into his viewing room to see my films. The machine had been focused on my pelvis. I could easily see my pelvic structures in detail. I was pleased that all seemed in order. I saw no evidence of cancer penetrating the prostate capsule. In fact I saw no evidence of cancer anywhere! The radiologist pointed out some smudges in the interior of my prostate gland, which could be the cancer. He was quick to add that they could also just be blood clots from my recent biopsy.

Then came his verdict: "Your prostate is a touch enlarged. This is a good study, and I don't see anything that looks like cancer outside your prostate!"

Thank God!

Of course I realized that for all its sophistication, the MRI would not see any microscopic spread of my cancer, but so far, so good. I thanked my God again as I headed for the Nuclear Medicine Department. Once again I was about to experience high-tech imaging, a bone scan.

————◄•••••••••————

Prostate cancer has an affinity for spreading to the skeleton. A bone scan will find it, sometimes years before an x-ray shows anything. The technology is impressive. It all begins with a radionuclide produced in a fission reactor. These radionuclides are unstable. Their decay releases gamma photons. Think of gamma photons as

83

light particles beyond our visual spectrum that can shine through a patient's body. A scanning camera, using sodium iodide crystals, can photograph this light.

The trick is getting a radionuclide into the bones. Technetium-99 will do that. This is a radionuclide bound to Phosphate, a basic ingredient of bone. When injected into a body, it is rapidly incorporated into the entire skeleton. Those bones begin to glow with the light of gamma photons. When our special camera looks at such a patient, it sees a glowing skeleton. The picture is a bit fuzzy, because the rest of the body is blurring the image. Bony areas of high metabolic activity glow even brighter. Prostate cancer metastatic to bones will produce such a hot spot.

I was aware that I would receive an injection of a radioactive isotope. The thought made me uncomfortable. My body would absorb about one Rad of radiation from the study. That's about three times what we each absorb annually from background radiation. The information would be worth the radioactive risk.

As a physician I had grown accustomed to balancing risk versus benefit. I knew that there was virtually always risk involved in diagnostic studies, treatments and medications. I suspect that a reasonable person would hesitate to take aspirin, if he were aware of all the potential problems it could cause.

I knew that I had entered a new world. In the dense underbrush of cancer, things were to become ever more risky. Here the new benchmark is the risk of dying a slow painful death of prostate cancer. Radioactive isotopes pale in comparison.

The actual process of the bone scan wasn't so bad. I arrived early at the Nuclear Medicine Laboratory for my injection. The Technetium 99 needs about two and a half hours to find its way to the bone. The therapist was wearing rubber gloves as he handled the lead container. Now that impressed me! He injected the medicine into the vein of my right arm. Then I had time to kill.

I hung out at the hospital, ate lunch, and had my chest x-ray done. Two and a half hours later I was lying on the scanning table staring at a huge camera that was staring back at me. It took about fifteen minutes for the camera to scan me from head to toe, and I was done.

Dr. Richard Budenz was the radiologist that day. I wandered into his viewing room and noticed my pictures on his view screen. There I was—a glowing skeleton staring into the room with my best Halloween grin. I noticed a hot spot in the middle of my right arm. No worry! That was where the Technetium-99 had been injected. I had noticed such an artifact on many previous films. Then my heart sank. I saw a definite hot spot in my skull! Trying to look calm, I pointed it out to Richard. He asked me:

"Mike, have you had any dental work done lately?"

"Of Course! That's it!" I crowed. "I had a new crown

85

and bridge a month ago!" The hot spot was right where my new choppers were to be found.

Then Richard said what I had been hoping to hear: "You're A-OK, Michael. I don't see anything abnormal."

There was no evidence of cancer in my bones! It was time to go home and open a bottle of bubbly. Richard shook my hand in warm congratulations.

"You know, Mike, I see you as a trail blazer for the rest of us. I know that I have about one chance in nine of going through the same thing. I'm counting on you to sniff out the very best therapy and show us that it isn't so bad."

Somehow I found that an encouraging picture. It was a sunny day in Cancerland, and now I was to be a trail-blazer through its murky forest.

I asked Richard what he knew about treating prostate cancer. He told me he had helped in a study using microwave radiation to destroy the cancer. The results had been disappointing. Otherwise he had little experience with prostate cancer.

He then told me, "Look up Seth Rosenthal at the Radiation Oncology Center. He really knows his stuff. He will give you some good advice about all your options, including radiation therapy."

I left the hospital with hope in my heart. *I could win this battle.* This cancer might truly be localized. I was eager to go home to share the good news with my family, but first I should call Dr. Rosenthal.

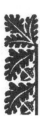

CHAPTER 9

HAVE YOU CONSIDERED RADIATION THERAPY?

I was surprised how accessible Seth Rosenthal was on the phone. I briefly told him my story. He said, "You sound like you need to talk. I would like to be available to a colleague in need. Can you come over in about an hour?"

Why not? I wasn't really mentally prepared to deal with this cancer any more today, but I knew this was an offer I didn't want to spurn. I accepted his invitation and was on my way in a few minutes.

The Radiation Oncology Center is a new hillside facility overlooking the community of Cameron Park. As I crossed its threshold, I felt unease in my gut. It reminded me of what I felt entering the Cancer Ward for my first time as an intern. I'd never expected to inhabit such a place. Feeling strangely embarrassed, I signed in at the window and waited.

I wasn't having much luck distracting myself with a three-month old magazine. Memories of cancer patients I cared for as a young doctor flooded into my consciousness. I was an Intern at Wilford Hall USAF Medical Center, Lackland Air Force Base, Texas. This is a busy military referral center, with patients flying in daily from all over the world. I began my two months training on the

Cancer Ward with trepidation. Little did I realize that those two months would be among the most dynamic of my professional life.

I'll never forget my orientation by a fellow intern. He had just completed two months of oncology and was moving on. We were sitting in a small office, discussing his patients, whom I would soon inherit. We discussed a young man afflicted with a rare form of leukemia. My colleague advised me, "The professors are excited about this patient. They're publishing a paper related to his care. Don't let this guy die, if you want a good evaluation on this service."

We discussed a middle-aged woman with end-stage leukemia. She had been supported for the past few months with transfusions of various blood products with diminishing success. Then he said, "The transfusions aren't working anymore. The attending physicians plan to stop her transfusions. She's going to die. You'll have to tell her tonight after evening rounds."

My first patient off the Medical Evacuation Plane late that evening was a young woman with newly diagnosed acute leukemia. She didn't realize how sick she was and needed urgent therapy in the morning. She had learned of her diagnosis just that morning at a New England air force base. She was put on a plane to Texas with little time to pack her clothes and say a few good-byes. She arrived on my ward about midnight in a state of emotional disarray, to say the least. As we talked, she broke down and cried! I was in a state of near exhaustion myself. I had spent the day attempting to learn the complex medical stories of 12 patients I had inherited that day. Somehow I managed to find the energy to sit up with this woman for a couple of hours—comforting her and attempting to banish her fears with the light of knowledge.

Later that night I found time for a nap before morning rounds. I remember lying on my bunk in the "on call room" thinking that this was going to be a challenging two months. Here we were making life and death decisions daily. Here people were looking the Grim Reaper in the face, and making him blink! I had been impressed with the resilience of the human spirit that day.

By the end of my two-month rotation, I had acquired the bare rudiments of skill in helping a patient die with dignity. My life's philosophy had been dramatically altered. I had accepted death as an inevitable part of living. As a young man in the prime of my life, I vaguely knew that it applied to me too, but I could push that off to a distant future.

<hr/>

Well doctor, the future has arrived. As I sat in the waiting room, I noticed a man in a wheelchair. A woman—I assume his wife—was pushing him into the room. He looked miserable. I could tell he was chronically ill. Physicians learn to recognize that look, but there was another look about him that disturbed me. There was panic on his face. I perceived it easily, probably because I was feeling it myself. His only words were to his wife, "Let's get out of here." He was wiping tears from his face as she wheeled him out the door. Oh Great! The first patient I see in this place is wheelchair-bound and in a state of apparent desperation—panic writ large on his face. How many of these souls are there in the bowels of this building, and where is my place among them?

Calling my name, a nurse appeared in the hallway. I mentioned, "That man seemed very agitated."

She whispered, "He just got some pretty bad news."

We entered an exam room where I went through the ritual of disrobing, weighing in, and vital signs. I thought I was looking like a fairly cool customer until the nurse asked me if I had high blood pressure. My blood pressure was higher than I had ever seen it. My body had betrayed me and announced the tension I was feeling.

I told her, "It looks like you've found me out. I'm nervous."

She smiled reassuringly and said, "We'll try it again when you've settled down."

She left me alone in the room with my magazine.

It wasn't long before Seth Rosenthal M.D. entered the room. He was a big man with an imposing presence. He quickly put me at ease and turned to business. After he took my medical history and performed his physical exam, he invited me to dress and join him in the conference room.

As I entered the room, Seth greeted me with the news, "Before I say anything else, I want to tell you that you have a curable cancer."

"Thanks for the good tidings!"

"You're welcome." Then he added, "Any physician would like to have you as his patient. You can make his numbers look good. In fact, I suspect that any therapy you choose will be successful. I would ask you to give some consideration to radiation therapy."

"Is that your recommendation?"

"I can cure you, but I need to tell you that the conventional wisdom today still insists that you should have a prostatectomy. That seems to be the standard therapy for men your age with your stage of cancer. You have no physical problems that would make surgery risky for you. Some physicians believe that long-term control rates—10 to 15 years after therapy—are somewhat better with surgery than with radiation therapy."

Now that was a nice mixed message! I think I just heard him say that he could cure me and would like the chance, but I should go somewhere else! I was determined to explore radiation therapy before I was sent back to the surgeons. I pressed on with my questions. I asked him exactly what radiation therapy would entail.

"You would receive 36 treatments, Monday through Friday, over a course of about seven weeks. You get to rest over the weekends. The treatments take about ten minutes each. You'd be out the door in about half an hour every day. We could give you a standing appointment every weekday, and then you could get on with your work."

"Would I feel any side effects?"

"Some people complain of fatigue about half way

through the therapy. Frankly, I think much of it is psychological."

Then he added, "You need to know that there are potential side effects. Your rectum and bladder will both receive radiation and can suffer damage—sometimes severe. Most men notice a definite change in their bowel habits, usually a change from one bowel movement daily to two. Some report a tendency towards loose stools. A small percentage develop bloody stools, usually about a year afterward. That can be controlled with cortisone enemas. Some men develop an inflamed bladder, a radiation cystitis, and seem to endure about six months of frequent or uncomfortable urination. The cystitis can be permanent. There are medicines that can help control those symptoms as well. It is possible to suffer complete loss of bladder or bowel control. Fortunately, that is rare."

I had not come to this session unprepared. I had some statistics in my hip pocket. I had read a journal reporting interviews of Medicare patients. These men had all chosen radical prostatectomies for prostate cancer. Their numbers were grim. Thirty-one percent of these men reported urine incontinence and were wearing diapers or pads daily. Twenty-three percent dripped urine "more than a few drops daily." Six percent underwent additional surgery for incontinence, and twenty percent had to have some form of medical treatment for stricture of the urethra.

The numbers describing impotence were equally grim. Ninety percent of the men described themselves as potent prior to surgery. After surgery, sixty-one percent reported "no full or partial erections." Only eleven percent had enjoyed erections firm enough for intercourse in the previous month! I was aware that these were all Medicare men, which meant most were sixty-five years or older. That age group would have worse statistics than mine. I didn't find that very comforting.

I knew that radiation therapy can cause its own sexual problems. The nerves controlling erection are right there in the capsule of the prostate. They get caught in the crossfire and can suffer radiation damage. It's hard to find credible post-therapeutic figures on impotence. The literature is so unreliable. To start with, men seem unreliable when asked about their sexual capacity.

I remarked to Seth, "I've heard that if surgeons were honest, they would be reporting impotence rates of at least 50%. I've also heard that radiation therapy can destroy erectile function, just like surgery."

"That's right. Some surgeons consider 'potency' one serviceable erection a year. You can imagine that their numbers look pretty good! A man's sexual capacity falls off with age anyway, so I have to factor a man's age into any odds I give. You're still pretty young; you can expect to find yourself on the low side of the averages. We report about 30% to 40% impotence. That's permanent! There's another group of men that manage to have regular intercourse, but report a definite decline in their ability to perform. Their erections are not as firm, nor as lasting."

I was becoming intensely aware that my sexual life might soon be over. I reassured myself: "No, that's not exactly right. My ability to have sexual intercourse, as I enjoyed it in the past, might be coming to an end. That doesn't have to be the end of my sexuality."

I had counseled a paraplegic once about his sexuality. It had been a brief discussion at his bedside in a busy emergency department. I had forgotten about the conversation. I met him again a few years later, and he greeted me with enthusiasm.

"Doc, thanks for giving me back my sexuality. Your advice was right on!"

Mystified, I asked him, "What did I say that struck such a chord in your heart?"

"You told me that I had to think of myself as a sexual creature. If I didn't see myself as deserving of love and sex, certainly no one else would."

He was right. Now it was my turn to learn from my patient. I could continue to be a sexual man. I would find some way to express that sexuality. In fact, I suspect that the physicians offering various appliances were unnecessary. They permitted a semblance of intercourse. If left alone, most couples would find a way to express their sexuality—to pleasure one another—without them.

I had to accept that impotence might be the price of a passport out of the desolate wilderness of cancer, which seemed to have barbed wire at all its borders. I remembered an elderly priest I once knew. I asked him if he had found his celibate life difficult. He replied, "The first seventy years seem to be the hardest."

"Well, how old are you?"

He smiled, "I just celebrated my seventieth birthday."

What an old joke. I should have seen it coming!

———————

But I had to concentrate on the conversation at hand. I had so many questions of Dr. Rosenthal.

"What about implanting radioactive seeds into my prostate? How does that compare with what you are offering me?"

Seth told me that such therapy wasn't available locally, but he would be happy to refer me to the people in Seattle who were doing such therapy.

He added, "You would be a good candidate."

I had heard about hormone suppression therapy. Physicians have long known that prostate cancer could be controlled by hormone manipulation, at least temporarily. Over fifty years ago Charles B. Huggins, working at the University of Chicago, discovered that androgens (male hormones) can dramatically stimulate the growth of prostate cancer. Withdrawing those same androgens slowed its growth. For that work he was awarded the Nobel Prize in Medicine. A man's testicles are his predominant source of androgen, most of which is testosterone. (His adrenal glands produce another ten percent of his androgens.) One surefire way to eliminate ninety percent of a man's androgen production is to remove his testicles! Castrating a man can prolong his life—sometimes for many years. Although it is becoming less common, castration is still practiced today in the battle against prostate cancer. The procedure is usually reserved for men with metastatic prostate cancer.

When cancer finds its way to a man's bones, especially the spine, pain can be overwhelming. Castration can provide dramatic pain relief. Unfortunately, the cancer eventually breaks free of these hormonal restraints and resumes its relentless growth. That may take two to five years, sometimes longer. I hoped that I would never need to make such a decision.

Estrogen was used for many years to interfere with the actions of testosterone. It had its own list of undesirable side effects, including growth of a man's breasts. Modern medicine now has new drugs to suppress testosterone production. One injection of a drug such as Lupron will stop the testicles' production of testosterone—sometimes for months. It's as effective as castration.

The new euphemism is "chemical castration!" I shuddered the first time I saw that in print. That's something else we need to remove from the medical lexicon. What patient wants to think of himself as castrated, be it chemically or otherwise?

The really big news? **Evidence is gathering that hormone suppression makes radiation or surgical therapy even more effective**. In this case two plus two equals five—possibly much more!

I asked Seth, "I've heard that hormonal suppression can improve my chances for survival. Nick has recommended monthly injections of Lupron. Would you recommend such therapy while undergoing radiation?"

"Absolutely. The Lupron will stop androgen production in your testicles. I would add Eulexin to block the effects of the last ten percent produced by your adrenal glands."

Seth looked at his watch. "You can take your time making your decision. I would recommend that you give yourself a month to decide. Then you'll have to move on this. I have some literature for you to review, and we'll talk about this again after you've had a chance to read it. I recommend that you talk to as many physicians as you can before you make your decision. You may want to call one of the Seattle physicians doing the seed implants. There are several local physicians who deal with prostate cancer every day. You need to look them up." He gave me a list of several physicians and I said my good-byes.

———————

On the way home I felt bewildered by the day's events. It had been a productive day. After months of inertia, I had finally begun to move on this problem. Medicine's most sophisticated imaging studies had failed to find any spread of my cancer. I had just left an interview with an expert, who anticipated a cure. As I reviewed the events of the day, I knew that I should be encouraged.

Somehow I wasn't. There remained too many unknowns, and certainly no guarantees. I tried to imagine what it would feel like to lie under a beam of x-rays for the first time, let alone for thirty-six times. What would it feel like to slowly destroy part of my body over seven weeks, an organ that had been a vital aspect of my adult life? I still had an abundance of investigation to do. It seemed overwhelming. I decided to just let go of it all and sleep on the matter. Perhaps in the morning my path would be more obvious.

⎯⎯••●●●●●●••⎯⎯

I was so distracted by the background noise of life for the next two days, that I didn't even try to deal with my cancer. That evening I settled into a couch with the literature Seth had given to me.

The first article was entitled "External Beam Radiation Treatment for Prostate Cancer: Still the Gold Standard." It was written by a prominent radiation specialist, Gerald E. Hanks, M.D. In the article, Dr. Hanks compares **X-ray therapy** (external beam radiation) to radical prostatectomy. He makes the bold statement that for a patient with early prostate cancer such as mine, survival rates for either therapy are essentially the same. He presents a series of 104 such patients. In his series, the cancer patients actually lived longer than the average American without prostate cancer! Could it be because of the close medical attention they received? *Meanwhile 87% of the men treated with external beam radiation were alive and clinically free of cancer in ten years.* Among the patients who died, only 14% died of their cancer. The majority of the deaths were unrelated to their cancer.

Dr. Hanks addressed one of the big problems in dealing with prostate cancer statistics.

"Because of the curious biology of prostate cancer, however, we must look at 10 or 15 year results in order to draw conclusions about the value of a specific treatment. This means that we are always half a generation behind when we compare the results of the best treatments used 10 or 15 years ago, with what we are actually doing now."

Radiation therapy has improved a great deal in the past 15 years. Obviously we won't have comparable studies for another 15 years.

To do a proper study, a large number of patients would have to be assigned randomly to either surgery or radiation—virtually a toss of the dice. A large association of medical centers, The Southwest Oncology Group, attempted to do that in 1990. They had to abandon the effort. After two years, they had enrolled only eight patients. We men are reluctant to let Lady Luck pick our therapy.

I read a review of Dr. Hank's article, written by E. David Crawford, M.D. He is Professor and Chairman of the Division of Urology, University of Colorado. He laments the "physician bias" in any article, including Dr. Hank's. He quoted a survey done in Toronto. Physicians were asked what therapy they would select, if they were stricken with prostate cancer:

"In this review, radiation therapists...almost uniformly stated that they would accept only radiation therapy if they had localized prostate cancer. Urologists chose the surgical route."

Cancer specialists, who were neither surgeons nor radiation therapists, were split between the two treatment modalities.

Dr. Crawford offered his own statistics for complications of radical prostatectomy:

> In our series, 1% of patients have experienced total (urine) incontinence, and 8% stress incontinence. (They leak urine when they cough or strain.) Rectal injury has not occurred. Return of sexual function is dependent on the patient's age and the stage of his tumor; 72% of the men under the age of 70 undergoing this procedure maintain their sexual potency.

He makes the points:

> There is no substantial data bank of patients followed 10 years after radiation therapy alone. The complications of radiation therapy parallel those of radical prostatectomy, though the major side effects, such as impotence and incontinence take longer to develop than the immediate effects seen after radical prostatectomy.

What's a mother to do? It was becoming obvious that I wasn't going to find consensus in the medical literature.

The final blow came when I read a report by the American Urological Association. They convened a panel of eleven experts to review the medical literature and publish recommendations for therapy. The objective was to settle this issue once and for all! These eleven physicians did yeoman's service. They reviewed 12,501 reports, comparing various therapies for prostate cancer. (I doubt that the average physician reads 12,501 articles in a life-time.) They were especially interested in how well patients fared at 5, 10, and 15 years.

The results? They "found the data inadequate for valid comparisons of treatments. Differences were too great among treatment series with regard to such significant characteristics as age, tumor grade, and pelvic lymph node status."

Basically they gave up! In the end the panel published recommen-dations for treatment options:

Options for management of localized prostate cancer include radical prostatectomy, radiation therapy, and surveillance. Radiation therapy includes external beam and interstitial treatments (seed implants)...**data from the literature do not provide clear-cut evidence for the superiority of any one treatment**.

I was especially intrigued by the next two recommen-dations:

Based on the panel's interpretation of the literature, and on their expert opinion, the patient most likely to benefit from radical prostatectomy would have a relatively long life expectancy, no significant surgical risk factors, and a preference to undergo surgery...

The patient most likely to benefit from radi-

)n therapy would have a relatively long life
)ectancy, no significant risk factors for radi-
)n toxicity, and a preference for radiation
therapy.

So what did they say? You pay your money, you make
your choice! Basically, if you think as a patient that you
might prefer surgery, go for it, and vice versa.

*If the combined wisdom of these men couldn't make
sense of the competing therapies, how the hell could I?*
Actually I found this quite liberating in a perverse sort of
way. I was now convinced that I wasn't going to find the
answer in the literature. It was a grand excuse to ease off
and listen to my intuition, to hear what my heart was
saying.

Both of my parents have recently been through radiation therapy. My father received radiation therapy for his
prostate cancer at age 78 a few years ago. My mother
developed laryngeal cancer and recently completed radiation therapy to her throat. She lost her voice in the process; we could no longer communicate by phone. I had
written several letters attempting to keep everyone
informed of my progress. My parents never responded. I
found that odd. They, especially, should understand what
I might be going through. I began to wonder if they had
even received the letters. It was time to call Dad and seek
his advice. I wanted to know what his experience had
been.

I was flabbergasted by his response, when I mentioned my cancer. There was irritation in his voice as he

said, "Michael, you've got to stop calling everybody and telling them you've got cancer. You're upsetting your mother, your brothers, and all your relatives in New Jersey. This is just something we men get as we get older, and you have to deal with it. Go get your x-rays like I did, and you'll be OK."

I tried again: "Dad, I'm not sure I want to have radiation therapy. I'm looking for a way get rid of this for the next thirty years."

"They gave me a certificate when I finished my therapy that says I'm cured. Look at me, I'm doing just fine."

I dropped the subject. I suppose that for someone who has been through the Great Depression and World War, prostate cancer is just a bump on the highway of life. But there was more, much more, in his response. This was a father uncomfortable with his child's illness. The real message here was that my parents couldn't deal with still another cancer in the family, especially involving their son. I understood that this was a topic to avoid in the future.

I couldn't imagine what my father's certificate was all about. I doubted that any physician was willing to certify his work with a guarantee. There are no guarantees in an oppressive land like cancer.

CHAPTER 10

IT'S OK TO CRY.

The idea of implanting radioactive particles in the prostate is not new. Physicians have been at it for almost a century. It's an attractive idea: put the radioactive source right into the cancer you're trying to kill. Therapists coined the word **brachytherapy** for this remedy. As early as 1911 Pasteau tried inserting a radium pellet up the penis of patients with prostate cancer. He used a catheter to place the pellet in the urethra where it passes through the prostate gland. Denning adopted the technique, and published a study involving one hundred patients about ten years later. His results were not encouraging. The cancers were stalled only temporarily, and he had significant problems with complications of therapy. Barringer tried implanting radium needles in 1917 with similar temporary results.

Radioactive implants fell into disrepute after that until 1972, when doctors tried again. This time physicians used isotopes such as iodine-125 in "seeds" which were implanted through large needles. The seeds, left in place permanently, gradually released their radiation, and became inert. The physicians implanted the isotopes surgically—actually opening the patients' abdomens, and directly visualizing their prostate glands. It turned out that this wasn't as easy as it may seem. I can only imagine what it must have been like; trying to work in the cramped, bloody environment of a man's pelvis, especially if the man were obese, with a deep narrow pelvis. It was difficult to get the uniform placement of seeds needed. Without uniform seed placement, the radiation dosage would be haphazard throughout the prostate. As might be expected, long term control of the cancers was not good, except for very early cancers.

In the late 1980's we had a breakthrough, as newer technologies came to the rescue. Physicians began to use ultrasound imaging to see where the needles were going. **Ultrasonography** uses sound waves of such high pitch that we can't hear them. The reflected echoes are gathered to form images by a computer. It's not such a new idea. Bats have been doing it for millions of years.

CAT scanning and ultrasound made it possible to accurately assess the size and shape of the prostate gland. Physicians could then plan the pattern of seed placement to insure uniform radiation dosages. The calculations are complex, but computers made them feasible. Finally physicians began placing the needles through a man's perineum (that patch of skin lying between a man's scrotum and rectum). A major surgical procedure was no longer necessary to place the seeds.

When I found an article by Dr. John C. Blasko, he had been doing such seed implants at the Northwest Tumor Institute since 1988. He treated 138 men with early prostate cancer with iodine-125 seeds. Ninety-three percent of them had no clinical evidence of cancer five years later. This really caught my attention! I contacted Dr Blasko's office and spoke to his nurse, Alea. She offered to send more information.

I wrote a letter to Dr. Blasko, outlining the details of my cancer. As I wrote my letter, the thought struck me: "He might not want me for a patient! What if I fell outside of his treatment criteria? It seemed that he was dealing primarily with early cancers. Was mine early enough? What would I do if he refused to accept my case?"

His article did not mention hormone suppression, so I assumed that he was not using such therapy. I could understand the reasons for that. Accepting patients on various hormone therapy might confuse the issue, making the results difficult to interpret. I decided to postpone any decision to start hormone suppression until I spoke to Dr. Blasko.

———— • ————

I was busily at work one evening when a cardiologist, Dr. Edmund Lee, dropped in for a chat. He expressed his concern about my health.

"I heard about your cancer. How are you holding up?"

"About as good as can be expected, I guess."

"You know, there was an article in Fortune magazine a few months ago by a fellow—I think he's the C.E.O. of Intel—who had prostate cancer. He went to Seattle for radiation therapy. It looked pretty positive. Would you be interested if I could find the article?"

"You bet I would! I've just been corresponding with a

doc up there about the same thing."

Ed committed to search for the article as he left, and the event passed my mind.

⎯⎯•••••⎯⎯

The next day I was eating breakfast in a coffee shop, as I enjoyed a lazy morning off duty. Someone had left the Wall Street Journal on the table, and I was idly looking it over. A large advertisement from Loma Linda University Medical Center caught my eye. They were advocating a new type of therapy for prostate cancer: **proton radiation**. My first reaction was emotional. "My God, can't a man even settle down with a newspaper without being reminded that he has cancer!?"

As my ardor cooled, I became fascinated by the thought of proton beam therapy. To create a beam of protons, the therapists at Loma Linda would need a cyclotron —an atom smasher! The ad didn't give much detail, but it offered a phone number I will never forget: 1-800-PROTON.

I called the number that morning. I was greeted by a pleasant receptionist who agreed to send some literature, and then offered to put me on the line with a financial specialist. He would help complete the paperwork for my insurance company. I respectfully declined, telling her that I'd wait for the info in the mail.

⎯⎯•••••⎯⎯

The next day as I arrived at work, I found a note from Edmund Lee with the promised article from *Fortune* magazine. It was written by Andy Grove and appeared in

Fortune's May 12, 1996 issue. I was mesmerized as I read the account of his prostate cancer. His cancer was picked up on a PSA screening exam, with numbers much like mine. He focused his considerable skills and resources on investigating every avenue of therapy. He was also impressed by the Partin Tables and realized that he was at risk. There was a substantial chance that his cancer was extending through his prostate's capsule. His initial impression?

"Clearly surgery did not cure everyone, even under the best conditions... The reports of incontinence and impotence...certainly motivated me to examine other types of treatment."

Mr. Grove began to consider "combination radiation"—external beam radiation combined with radioactive seeds. The theory is that the seeds can deliver a potent dose directly to the tumor contained in the prostate gland. External beam radiation can effectively destroy any cancer that has escaped the capsule with a lesser dose of radiation than would be necessary to penetrate the entire prostate gland. Hopefully, the side effects of radiation would be kept to a minimum.

Andy Grove finally concluded:

> PSA has only been around for ten years, so as far as I was concerned, both surgery and radiation had relevant data for only ten years or less, and not much even at ten years. But it occurred to me that if combination radiation, which looked better to me than external radiation by itself, only gave me ten years of

freedom from disease, I could buy myself a ten-year reprieve from disease relatively inexpensively, considering that it's a lot less onerous treatment.

Andy had hope that another breakthrough would happen during that ten-year reprieve, as he traveled to Seattle for his brachytherapy. His therapy was a bit different than that offered by John Blasko. The seeds were so hot, that they were only temporarily left in place.

Mr. Grove offered advice which rang true to me: *"I think you should hit a tumor with what you believe is your best shot, early and hard."* He then added:

> In my case, it was a combination of hormones, high-dose-rate implant radiation, and external beam radiation. For others like Senator Dole and General Schwarzkopf, it was surgery. If my best friend had this disease, my advice to him would be, 'Investigate, choose, and do—and do it quickly. Be aggressive now. Don't save the best for later.'

As for me, I was greatly encouraged. If it was good enough for the C.E.O. of Intel, it was good enough for me! I was looking for more than a ten-year reprieve, but I'd take what I could get. The fog of confusion was beginning to clear in the wilderness. I began to think increasingly in terms of radiation therapy, especially as offered in Seattle.

I found the promised mailing from Loma Linda University Medical Center in my mailbox the next day. It included a short video, entitled *The Convergence of Science, Medicine, and Engineering*, showing smiling patients laying their bodies upon treatment tables for various cancers. It presented a brief discussion of the underlying physics and theory of proton therapy.

The attached literature was much more interesting. My suspicions were confirmed. Loma Linda has installed a cyclotron with a three story, 95 ton gantry designed to focus a fine beam of heavy particles (protons) onto a patient's cancer. They explain, at least theoretically, how the beam can deliver the majority of its energy into the heart of the cancer, avoiding the surrounding healthy organs. I hungrily devoured the statistics. They looked pretty good! The project became operational in 1990. That gives them a relatively short track record, which concerned me.

I asked Seth Rosenthal what he thought about proton beam therapy. He had obviously thought about this question before. His answer came quickly.

"There are some intriguing theoretical reasons why this should be better than what I offer, but I'm not so sure their numbers are any better than mine. Perhaps I'm just a bit envious that I don't have my own cyclotron to play with, but I don't think they bestow any great advantage upon the patient."

I had learned to trust Seth's opinion. I knew he was a competent physician who stayed abreast of developments. He would have carefully evaluated any alternative forms of radiation therapy. I considered him honest enough to tell me if he thought Loma Linda offered any therapeutic advantage. I took his word for it.

I saw one major disadvantage with going to Loma Linda: I would have to go to Loma Linda! I would have to find an apartment in the area, and live there for a couple months while undergoing therapy. Once again I was faced with the prospect of lost work for a prolonged time, with the added expense of living half way between Los Angeles and Palm Springs. I would have to leave my family and support system during a critical time, when I really needed them. It all seemed a bit overwhelming to contemplate, especially when the advantage may be only minimal. Even though I was attracted to the concept of proton therapy, I relegated it to second place. My eyes were still on Seattle.

I took the time to once more consider "watchful waiting." I actually found a posting on the Internet by Bart Moran, a man with prostate cancer who chose that option. I was a bit amazed when I read his numbers. He was diagnosed with prostate cancer at the relatively young age of 57. He had stage B cancer, Gleason Score 5, and PSA 8.4. All his numbers were equal to, or better than mine. Conventional wisdom certainly considered him curable; yet he chose to avoid seeking a cure. He was convinced that the risks and complications of aggressive therapy outweigh the potential of cure. He was chagrined by the sequence of events that follow discovery of an elevated PSA.

When a doctor says, "You have cancer," ...

112

fear obliterates reason. The doctor's not in the same space. The odds are he doesn't have cancer, and wants to get on with his job of treating illness without putting too much weight on some of the more 'subtle' side effects of treatment—like erections and bladder control.

Mr. Moran was skeptical that most therapeutic interventions were of much use. He considered our success rate unacceptable. He quoted statistics asserting that we have not changed the overall survival rate in thirty years. His theory was that our bodies could better endure this indolent cancer without the assault of modern therapies.

About a third of the time when the tests show that the cancer is confined, it's actually spread outside of the prostate to surrounding tissue or bones, and isn't curable with the treatment they usually recommend—i.e. radical surgery.... the 'big C' in prostate cancer isn't as big as it is in most cancers, and that it usually grows very slowly.

He quoted Willet Whitmore from Sloan-Kettering: "Growing old is invariably fatal. Prostate cancer is only sometimes so."

It is important to emphasize that watchful waiting is not synonymous with doing nothing. Instead, it is a concept that accepts cancer as just another disease, much like arthritis, diabetes, or AIDS. All are capable of causing an untimely death. All can be stalled in their relentless progress.

113

Watchful waiting involves close medical observation, with periodic physical exams while following such parameters as PSA. Complications are dealt with as they arise. For example if the PSA begins to rise, the patient may then elect to have a prostatectomy, or receive a few months of hormone suppression. This is the opposite end of the spectrum from Andy Grove who advocated giving it "your best shot, early and hard."

Some advocates of watchful waiting recommend it for men as young as sixty. This might have been a good approach for my father, but sixty years seemed a bit young to me. A healthy man at sixty can reasonably hope to live another generation. In rebuttal, proponents of watchful waiting claim that our aggressive therapies have failed to prolong the lives of prostate patients. A recent study showed a continuing rise in the death rate for prostate cancer over six years. During that same time the USA saw a six-fold increase in the rate of prostatectomies.

I suspect a better age limit for watchful waiting is seventy years—unless a man has some over-riding illness threatening to cut his life short. Other factors to consider include the Gleason Score and clinical staging. The Gleason score is an attempt to predict the malignancy of a cancer; therefore, it would only make sense that a man would prefer to have a low score, if he selects watchful waiting. Early staging and a small tumor are definite pluses. These are, of course, the same parameters that provide the best chance of a cure.

I have seen the phrase "watchful doing" advocated in

the literature. That makes more sense to me. It carries a vague commitment to do something when the time is right. When is the right time? To quote the Great Bard, "Therein lies the rub." With the right numbers, that could be a few years—a few years avoiding the trauma, expense, disability, and complications of major surgery, radiation, etc.

Opponents of watchful waiting fear that the window of opportunity could slam shut while one pretends to be in purposeful activity. They claim that the numbers a man would use are inaccurate at best. No one really knows how his cancer is staged until the pathologist has the specimen in his hands. The Gleason Score can vary with the pathologist interpreting the specimen. The PSA can even vary from lab to lab.

———

I heard those people who were entreating me to wait—to preserve the quality of my life. I heard the sirens' call! Was one more year of normal sexuality worth the possible increased risk? How about two more years? I had absolutely no symptoms! It would have been easy to drift along doing nothing. Being a bit of a gambler, I could have hoped for another 5 to 10 years of a life without catheters, diapers, or impotence.

I'm reminded of the words of a patient with terrible Parkinson's Disease. I asked him how he felt about his illness. He commented, "You have to play the hand you've been dealt." The vexation is that sooner or later you have to show your cards. I suspected that I was not holding a full house. I was 54 years young. Intuitively, I doubted that I would make it into my eighties without going for a cure. My psyche seemed to need that hope of a cure, ephemeral as it may be. I relegated watchful waiting to somewhere near the bottom of my list.

One of the first therapies I investigated was cryosurgery—a process of freezing the prostate gland to kill the cancer. In the community of men with prostate cancer it is often referred to with the irreverent moniker of *"Ice Balls."* Physicians freeze the prostate by inserting multiple freezing probes into the gland. The urethra is protected with a warming catheter. The prostate is transformed into a ball of ice, with the freezing zone sometimes deliberately extended into the surrounding tissue, to kill any cancer that may have penetrated the capsule.

Ice Balls was my first hope. However, that optimism was short lived. Cryosurgery would not permit me to evade the surgeon's knife. My research convinced me that this procedure needed another ten years of refinement.

The therapy is so new that there is no track record. We don't know how cryosurgery patients will do in ten years.

Most patients are impotent after cryosurgery. It's the same never-ending conundrum: How does one kill the cancer growing around the nerves in the capsule without destroying the nerves as well? It does not matter whether the nerves are damaged by radiation, a surgeon's blade, or Ice Balls. The end result is impotence.

Katsuto Shinohara et. al. performed cryosurgery on

102 men for localized prostate cancer. They concluded:

> Cryosurgical ablation of the prostate can result in negative post-treatment biopsies and undetectable serum PSA levels. However it is associated with significant side effects, and the long term durability of the procedure is unknown... and patients must be so advised. Additionally, the procedure is associated with significant morbidity within the first few months of treatment. With improvements in technology, imaging, and freezing technique, the incidence of rectal injury is now low... but urinary retention has become a major problem.

Editorial comments by H. Ballentine Carter, Dept. Of Urology, Johns Hopkins University Medical School, were not very encouraging. He makes the point that biopsies taken after therapy will show living prostate cells. If cryosurgery does not destroy all the healthy cells in a prostate gland, he wonders how many cancer cells may also survive. Then he cautions:

> Finally cryosurgery is associated with morbidity. In this series urinary obstruction requiring transurethral resection (surgery) occurred in 23% of patients, stress incontinence in 15%, and impotence in 84% of men who were potent before cryosurgery...From this study and other recent evaluations of cryotherapy, the message that should be given when counseling patients is clear, that is cryosurgery is an experimental form of treatment with no proved benefit that is not risk free.

Fred Lee of the Dept of Radiology, Crittenton

Hospital joins in with his own editorial comments:

> A recurring theme in this and other reports on prostate cryosurgery is the search for technical considerations that could standardize and improve results from this procedure. Because of this uncertainty over exactly how cryosurgery of the prostate should be performed, I personally believe that the widespread clinical application of this procedure is premature.

Sadly, I put Ice Balls on the bottom of my list. It was becoming clear to me that if I chose to avoid surgery, my best chance of a cure would be with seed implants.

I tried to imagine what surgery would be like. I could easily accept the image of my entering the operating suite, surrounded by men and women I had known for years. I had no doubt that they would give me the best care they could muster. Contemplating the recovery period was the problematic part. That's when my mind would go into *TILT.* I just couldn't accept the prospect of enduring a catheter for weeks (months?) and missing work for months.

I tried talking to friends who had been through cancer surgery, any kind of cancer. Diane is a contemporary of mine, and went through a hysterectomy for uterine cancer at age 27. I can only imagine how traumatic that had been for her as a young woman. She surprised me with a question:

"Have you cried yet?"

The question seemed strange to my macho, male heart—almost irrelevant.

"No, I haven't. In fact, I've done everything I can to keep a cheerful attitude. Why do you ask?"

"Well, you will!" Her smile vanished. "That's when you will know that you are really dealing with your cancer. When it happens, just tell yourself that it's OK to cry."

In my quest for answers, I searched out one of my priests, Rev. Sanford Miller. He listened as I rambled on for perhaps fifteen minutes about searching for meaning in this illness, making the responsible choice in therapy, etc. When my ardor was spent, he asked me, *"Did you think you were going to live forever?"*

I was stunned into silence with that simple question. Then he added, "You are dealing with your own mortality. That's what is really happening here."

Yes! Of Course! He was right! I had buried my struggle over my mortality under piles of research papers, memos, magazine articles, and male bravado.

It should be so obvious to us all that we are mortal beings. No one has gotten off this planet alive. Even Jesus Christ had to die. Why does it come as such a surprise when we are diagnosed with a fatal disease?

The next day I was home alone and feeling terribly blue. I had gotten home at three AM from a difficult shift at the emergency department. I'm convinced that my destiny has me in that ER for a purpose. That place is like an anvil upon which I'm hammered from time to time. I've learned many a lesson of life in that forge.

Today was to bring yet another instruction for me. I felt as if my psyche had been scraped down to bedrock during last night's shift. In my sleep-deprived state, I knew that I would mope through the entire day, unless I tried to revive my spirits. A soak in the hot tub and a long nap were definitely what this doctor prescribed.

After an hour in the hot tub, I snuggled under the down comforter on our bed. This was definitely my comfort zone, but my melancholy persisted, unshakable. In fact it seemed that each time I shoved it down, it would bubble up with renewed vigor. I wasn't even sure why I felt so woebegone, but this was a grief that would not be denied!

I began sobbing uncontrollably. There didn't seem to be much I could do except to embrace my sadness; but this seemed so much more than sadness. I felt myself swept into an emotional vortex—a vortex of anguish, anx-

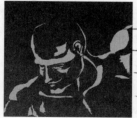

iety, despair, and anger! No! Not anger. It was *Rage*! Rage over the unfairness of it all. Rage that I had been stricken with cancer. Rage with the fierce sense of a broken covenant.

I suppressed a compelling urge to climb naked out of my bed, and throw a chair through the plate glass window—release this overwhelming passion.

when I thought of Diane's words:

"It's OK to cry!"

I surrendered to my grief. I haven't cried like that since I was a small child. I mean I really got into it—wailing, sobbing, cursing, complaining out loud. I must have lain there for half an hour—wallowing in self pity, soaking my pillow in tears—before I managed to fall asleep. I cried myself to sleep like a child, my emotions spent.

When I awakened, I felt reborn. I knew I had crossed a threshold. As I lay there contemplating what was happening to me, I thought about Rev. Miller's words and had a glimpse of what was going on. *I had been mourning the loss of my sense of immortality!* I realized that every one of us, facing cancer, has to go through this process. Probably every one of us facing any serious illness for the first time has to get through this stage.

Here was something I had sensed in my conversations with Patty and Diane. Here was a common bond linking all cancer survivors! Now I really understood what Diane was trying to say. This had been my initiation into the fraternity of cancer—a fraternity of men and women who had accepted their mortality. Many of these people had looked the Grim Reaper in the eye and made him blink. I felt like a dilettante in their company.

It was then that I knew my attitude towards life would be forever changed. We all need to wrestle with the Angel of Death, before we understand how precious life is. This is the gift cancer brings in its hands.

I began to think of life in shorter terms, to li

present. Retirement would take care of itself—if I was given the grace to live that long. I had already begun to savor each new day as a gift to be enjoyed. I thought of the first heart transplant patient I'd met. How courageous he had seemed to me at the time! He had truly looked the Grim Reaper in the eye. He greeted every morning with thankfulness, a bonus day. I hoped that I could approach the rest of my life, however long or short, with the same reverence and gratitude.

⬦⬦⬦⬦⬦⬦⬦

As I reflect back on my feelings then, I'm reminded of a wonderful play, *The Legacy*, by Mark Harelik. He has written a powerful scene in which a young mother is dying of cancer. She verbally accosts her rabbi with palpable anger and anguish. She demands that he explain why she is dying a slow, premature death. The rabbi points out that many people die gruesome, unfair deaths every day and answers her question with a question of his own: *"Did you think you were special?"*

That question will forever reverberate in my heart. Now I understand what that poor beleaguered rabbi was trying to say. Yes, I did think I was special. We all have the right to think of ourselves as unique, special souls.

My mother told me I was special every night, as she tucked me in. I spent much of my early childhood living in a house trailer, on the back of a carnival lot; yet my parents had convinced me that I was more than a "carny." They expected great things of me. I was special. I was the first born of a large third generation of Italian cousins. My grandmother made it clear that I was her favorite—special. I was the one who was going to go on to college. I led many of those cousins on to college. I was the first doctor. I was still serving at the altar in college at twenty-one years of age, still a virgin. You're damn right I thought I was special!

Cancer had taken that specialness away from me, with the force of a train wreck.

I wasn't immortal, and I wasn't special.

No one gets to be special in Cancerland.

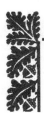

CHAPTER 11

CHEMICAL CASTRATION

In November the Fates decided to move me off the dime. It seemed as if every emergency shift I worked presented some poor soul who was suffering complications of prostate cancer.

One man was 91 years old. He arrived with pelvic pain, unable to urinate. His family knew that he had prostate cancer, but they refused to tell him. He was a bit senile, and I doubt he was fully capable of comprehending his illness anyway. His sons had been making his medical decisions for him, and they chose to treat him with watchful waiting.

As I palpated his abdomen, I realized that his bladder was markedly distended. No wonder he was so uncomfortable! It was obvious to me that his prostate cancer had now grown so large, that it pinched off his plumbing. His urethra was compressed as it passed through his cancerous prostate gland. I performed a rectal exam. With my finger in his rectum, I could feel that his prostate gland had been transformed into a huge, irregularly shaped cancerous mass, about the size of a grapefruit.

I managed to pass a narrow catheter up his penis and past the obstruction. When the catheter reached his ballooned bladder, it drained out a quart of urine. The poor man was so relieved that he wouldn't stop thanking me.

I advised his family that the catheter was only a temporary fix, and he would need further urological care. That's when his sons requested that I keep their secret. They were adamant. They did not want their father to know he had cancer.

This brought up all sorts of issues for me. Cancer still remains the unspeakable pestilence in many quarters. Don't say the word *"cancer,"* and we may avoid its grasp. Was I willing to join in this collusion?

I was in an ethical quandary. I believe in honesty with my patients. This man had a right to know what was happening to his body! It is possible to be honest without being brutally honest, but this concerned family wasn't going to hear my argument. Besides, who was I to force my ethical concepts upon these people? I chose the path of least resistance and quietly acceded to their request. I said nothing to this man about the beast lurking in his groin.

A few days later I was on duty when a 57-year old man presented with severe low back pain. You guessed it. He had far advanced prostate cancer that had spread to his pelvis and lumbar spine. When I reviewed his X-rays, I realized that his spine had several moth-eaten vertebrae. One was collapsing and causing his pain. Those pictures sent a shudder up my own spine. I actually had to take a short break after I admitted that man to the hospital.

That same week I cared for another man in his late fifties who was dying of metastatic prostate cancer. He was in constant, severe pain, despite huge doses of narcotics. The cancer was invading his bones. His spine was collapsing. He had become seriously anemic, weak, and thin. His cancer had transformed him from a robust man of 195 pounds to a character out of Dachau, in three years.

His right arm had broken that night as his son lifted him into bed. X-rays showed cancer invading his right humerus. I didn't have much to offer him except pain relief and a call to the orthopaedist.

I remember the orthopaedist shaking his head as he stared at the films and saying, "You know, Mike, I really have no idea how I'm going to fix this!"

My world was filling with men bearing prostate cancers, much more than I had been aware of over my thirty years of medicine. Was this just another baby buggy phenomenon? Was there a tidal shift happening in the world of prostate cancer? Was my guardian angel trying to tell me something?

My next shift was "graveyard"—midnight to eight in the morning. By four AM the department was uncharacteristically quiet. I was making plans to sneak a nap in the break room, when a car almost crashed through the ambulance entrance! An excited middle aged man burst into the department, announcing that his girlfriend was "dying of a stroke or something." We had no idea what to expect as we ran out to the car with a wheelchair.

What we found was a woman in the throes of a dramatic panic attack. She was breathing at fifty breaths a minute. Her hands and feet were convoluted in spasms. She was convinced she was dying!

After we moved her into a bed and calmed her, she told her story. Her fiancé had recently been diagnosed with prostate cancer. She had supper that evening with a prostate cancer support group, her first meeting. The focus of support that evening was the wife of a man with prostate cancer. Her husband had been admitted to the hospital with complications of end-stage cancer. He was dying.

My patient was overwhelmed with what she had heard that night. She was convinced that her fiancé was doomed. It would be her destiny to watch her beloved boyfriend die a horrible, painful death. She assumed that their sexual life was soon to be over. She was fearful of being left alone.

I took a risk and shared my own experience. A physician must be wary of revealing too much of himself to a patient. I've never been sure why, but I knew that I had to tell my own story that night.

I announced that I too had prostate cancer. I then declared that I had no intention of dying soon, nor of giving up my sexuality, nor of leaving my loved ones alone. This was a powerful revelation for them. It created an immediate bond among us. I was thankful that the night was slow, and we had time to talk. I had time to give them a fresh perspective on what they were facing. It was that night I heard myself saying that I was going to Seattle for seed implants.

After they left I reflected on that statement. I repeated it out loud. "I'm going to Seattle to have seed implants." Yeah, I think that's what I'm going to do! I resolved to contact Dr. Blasko in the morning.

As luck would have it, Dr. Blasko was booked up for months. He was moving to the University of Washington Cancer Center after a Christmas holiday break. I made the first available appointment in February. I felt uneasy about the delay and wasn't sure what I should do in the meantime.

<hr />

The next week I again immersed myself in the medical literature. I found an article explaining that patients with low PSA levels did the best after therapy—any therapy. That came as no surprise. What did surprise me was the author's statement that *the PSA is the single most important prognostic tool*—more important than Gleason Score, more important than clinical stage A versus B! There is a definite fall in survival rates for men with PSA values above twenty. In fact, the line was getting a bit shaky by fifteen!

Damn! It had been four months since I had tested my PSA and it was twelve then. One lab actually measured fifteen! My God! *Had I waited too long?* I really had to do something—and soon. I didn't even want to find out how high my PSA had risen by now.

I had to start hormone therapy as soon as possible. I had not discussed my therapy with Dr. Blasko. It was time to call Seattle again. Alea answered the phone. I told her that I couldn't wait until February. I needed to start hormone therapy. She sounded surprised.

"You mean you're not on hormone suppression therapy yet?"

"No, I assumed that Dr. Blasko wouldn't want me to do that without first discussing it."

She reassured me, "Most of his patients are on some sort of hormone suppression. He would have no objection at all. You should ask your urologist about starting Lupron." Suddenly I was feeling genuinely foolish! I had made the reckless assumption that Dr. Blasko would discourage my taking Lupron. For want of a simple phone call, I had let this cancer continue its sinister work completely unobstructed!

As I hung up the phone, I reflected upon my predicament. Here I stood as a physician with thirty years of medical training and experience, and I had made a foolish presumption that could jeopardize my care. Despite my conversations with multiple physicians, I did not get all the guidance I needed! Was this my fault or theirs? I forced down my rising anger and fear. It was suddenly eminently clear why patients can be so frustrated over lack of communication. It's one of the complaints I hear most frequently: "The doctor didn't keep me informed." I could see why a lay person would feel so vulnerable, and why he would need to pose vigilant questions throughout the perilous course of diagnosis and treatment.

Feeling dangerously behind the power curve, I called Nick Simopoulos' office, determined to get started on Lupron that day. *I hit a bureaucratic wall!*

Nick's receptionist informed me, "I will have to get authorization for Lupron therapy from your primary care doctor, Dr. Barnhill."

"How long will that take? Can we get authorization today?"

"I may be able to. I'll see what I can do and give you a call."

The rest of the morning seemed an eternity. By early afternoon I was in a near panic. I decided that I was going to do whatever it took to receive a shot of Lupron that afternoon! I called Nick's office again and asked his receptionist, "Have you had any luck with authorization process?"

She told me, "Dr. Barnhill is not authorized to approve Lupron therapy. Your care has been referred to a case manager in San Francisco. It will probably be a few days, maybe a week before we get authorization. I'll call you when I hear from them. Meanwhile I can pencil in an appointment for your shot next week."

"What if I pay for the shot myself? How much could it cost?"

"You wouldn't want to do that. The shots are about $500.00!"

Yea Gods! That stuff was expensive. She was right. I made an appointment for next week and hung up.

It didn't take me more than a few minutes to be in a stew again. I was feeling powerless, unable to move the bureaucratic machinery any faster than anyone else. I paced about the room for a few minutes in a near panic. I considered going to war with the insurance company. Call the president of the company! Call a lawyer! Call a state agency! I knew I wasn't thinking very clearly. I managed to calm down enough to call Nick directly.

"Nick! Help! I know this isn't logical, but I'm in a panic! I need to start Lupron ASAP. It will be forever before I can get official authorization. Is there anything you can do to help me?"

Nick was wonderful. He reassured me, "Come on over to the office today. We'll work something out."

God bless that man! I would have kissed him, if he had been within grabbing distance. I managed to arrive at his office before closing time. A few minutes later I had a shot of Lupron in my left buttock. Nick gave me a prescription for Eulexin tablets, and I headed for the pharmacy.

The Eulexin wasn't cheap either—$365.00 for a month's supply. It didn't take a great deal of math to realize that a man electing hormone suppression therapy would spend about $10,000.00 a year! How did the average American family afford this? For five years of therapy, we're talking about the price of a college education. No wonder my insurance company referred my care to a case manager.

And so it had started, with my first monthly shot of Lupron on November 25. I made a mental note that the next injection was due Christmas day. It had not been easy baring my buns to that nurse's needle, despite my panic. I knew I was crossing another threshold. I was now officially a patient with prostate cancer *on hormonal therapy*. I had picked a path at one of life's intersections. My path was beginning to narrow, and yet I felt a great sense of relief. I had subdued the beast—at least for a while.

Breathing room, how good it felt! Why had I waited so long?

Of course, I knew one answer to my rhetorical question: *because I had strong misgivings*. I had repeatedly found pessimistic literature. There are respectable people insisting that modern medicine has not prolonged the lives of men with prostate cancer. There is some glimmering that this may change with the new wave of early diagnosis. I was counting on that, as I started down the primrose path of medical intervention.

I was now chemically castrated! God, I hate that expression! The Lupron in my left buttock would stop all production of testosterone by my testicles—as if I had indeed been castrated. I actually went one step beyond that; I was also taking Eulexin (generic name Flutamide). This drug has the ability to block my body's use of any stray male hormones produced by my adrenal glands.

There are other drugs on the market that I could have taken. Most are variations on the same theme, all with their claims of superiority. I chose these because they had been around a while, and I had a better idea of the risks involved.

Nothing in this world seems to come without its price. I knew I would be impotent in a couple of months. I had read that my bones would begin to thin, raising the specter of osteoporosis in my old age, assuming I would have an old age. I knew I would begin to lose muscle mass and strength. It would be just a matter of days before the hot flashes began.

And of course, there is no guarantee. Some cancers just ignore any attempt to manipulate them with hormonal blockade.

I had heard of other possible side effects such as depression, fatigue, weight gain, and diarrhea. The implied promise was that this would all be temporary. Somehow I would endure them all in my search for a cure.

I tried to approach my changing physiology with a positive attitude. It would be interesting to see just what hot flashes were all about. God knows menopausal women have endured them since the dawn of time. I had been told that my impotence wouldn't be as troublesome as I imagined, because I would lose all interest in sex. That was hard for me to conceive. Could a few drops of daily testosterone have that much impact on such an integral part of who I thought I was?

—•••••••—

I had other friends advocating all manner of vitamins, food supplements, herbs, teas, enemas, therapeutic massage, acupuncture, meditations, Eurythmy, diets, exercises, art therapy, visualizations, and homeopathic remedies. They urged consultations with chiropractors, Anthroposophical physicians, homeopaths, faith healers, and mediums. One comrade urged me to consider a clinic in Mexico. Another pleaded with me to avoid radiation therapy at all costs. Alternative medicine is out there, alive and well—a multibillion dollar industry. All this well-meaning advice created a philosophical dilemma for me.

Here I was, a physician fully trained in the art of western medicine, and sick for the first time. All my training had reinforced the message: The true path to a cure lay within my profession. Now it was time to fish or cut bait.

My path to medicine has certainly not been conventional. Every carnival I remember had someone peddling the equivalent of snake oil. As a youth, I remember one particularly colorful gentleman, Doc Holiday. In retrospect, I suspect his moniker was based on the rumor that he carried a derringer in his boot. A man's name on a carnival midway frequently bears little resemblance to his birth certificate. I hadn't yet heard of the shootout at the OK Corral, so I missed the subtlety.

Doc Holiday was a charismatic speaker, who sold bottles of huge red pills. He virtually promised to make the Fountain of Youth unnecessary. I once watched in amazement as he held a crowd's rapt attention, while a million dollar, forth of July fireworks display was bursting over the midway. Now that's charismatic! There he stood "in the rockets' red glare"—claiming he was seventy years old, collecting ten dollars a bottle for his nostrum. Ten dollars could represent a day's wages when I was a youth.

I met Doc at the cookhouse a few days later. He was filling his pill bottles from a five gallon jug of huge red vitamin pills. He confided in me that he bought them from a discount house somewhere south of the border. Later, when I caught a peek at his driver's license, I realized he was forty-one years old!

So I *know* there are charlatans out there. There are also some well-meaning workers on the perimeter of medicine who are blazing new paths to health. Some are enlightened. Some are quacks. Frankly, I suspect some are delusional. Despite that conviction, I'm willing to accept that some have validity. I might even bet a week's wages on that. The problem is that we're not talking about a week's salary. We're talking about betting my life!

I certainly don't claim that conventional western medicine has all the answers. The history of my profession is replete with blind alleys and misguided therapy. Some of the most glaring examples included bleeding patients to cure them, or irradiating normal thymus glands in children.

Most people attempt to cover all bases. When ill, they accept what conventional medicine has to offer and then add a selection of alternative therapies as they see fit. If they're then fortunate enough to be cured, they give the lion's share of credit to the alternative care they elected. I have seen myself discounted as a physician several times in just such circumstances.

I especially remember a young woman with gonorrheal arthritis. (That's right! Gonorrhea can cause devastating arthritis!) One knee was so red hot, she couldn't walk. I hospitalized her for intravenous penicillin therapy. Her mother visited her three times a day with an herbal tea. When she left the hospital, she was walking normally. Guess who got the credit for her cure.

⸺•••••••⸺

I mulled over advice to take extra calcium and Vitamin D—to reduce bone thinning. I suspect it's more complicated than that. If hormone therapy causes bone to reabsorb and dump calcium into my bloodstream, then I already have high blood levels of calcium. That probably means that my kidneys are busy excreting calcium—attempting to keep blood calcium levels normal. I wasn't sure I wanted to compound the problem by taking calcium supplements. It seemed like a great way to form kidney stones, but of course that's all conjecture on my part.

I considered taking vitamin and food supplements, but I kept coming back to the same catch 22: "Do I really want to provide all the raw materials for rapid cell growth and repair, when I'm trying to kill cancer cells in my groin?"

I decided that the optimum therapy for me would embrace what I knew best. Mark Twain once said: "Put all your eggs in one basket, and then WATCH THAT BASKET." That would be my approach. My basket would be woven with strands of knowledge, knowledge that endured the light of careful scientific methods. I would carry that basket, as I picked my way through the perilous minefields of cancer.

I resolved to tuck my chin down and get through whatever the next year would bring—without vitamins, without supplements, and without alternative medicine. My fate would be in the hands of conventional medicine.

The next couple of months were good! I said that to Patty one night on the graveyard shift. She nodded in understanding, and added:

"That period of indecision you've been through was a tough phase! Therapy is the best phase. Now you're the center of attention. You have all the resources of medicine marshaled about you. You can feel like you're kicking that cancer in the ass!"

"Yeah," I agreed, "I see what you mean. I can imagine how good I will feel when I finish my therapy and walk out of the doctor's office for the last time."

"Wrong! That's the hardest! First of all there will be no last time."

She stopped to choose her words carefully.

"No one is ever going to tell you that you are cured."

Then she added, "For me, it felt as if I had been cut adrift—really alone. In my quiet moments, I still wonder if my cancer is coming back. I live from check-up to check-up. I will admit that I'm getting less paranoid as the years go by."

I asked if she had any advice for me as I went through my therapy.

"Yes, I do. I've found that it's good for me to help other women with breast cancer. You're in a unique position. You're both physician and patient! That gives you great power to comfort any man, woman, or child with cancer. It would be good for you."

The next day as I pondered that advice, I began to think about writing this book.

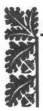

CHAPTER 12

DR. BLASKO, I PRESUME?

As the trip to Seattle approached, I began to feel uneasy. I tried telling myself that it would be good to get on with my therapy, to get my life back to normal. That didn't seem to help much. I looked up an old friend, Reverend Richard Lewis. Richard seemed to fathom the problem almost as I began speaking. (Am I that transparent?)

"Michael, this is typical behavior for a physician. You have spent thirty years of your life becoming the best possible doctor you can be. You have spent much of that time taking care of other people in a competent, professional manner, but you have always been in charge. This time you don't get to be in charge.

"You have carefully researched your options and chosen your therapy. You have picked good, competent physicians. Now it's time to let someone else take care of you. Put yourself in your physicians' hands, and let them do their job. You must learn to trust your colleagues, to trust your destiny, to trust your God."

Wonderful advice! Now I know how Atlas must have felt as the world was lifted from his shoulders. I realized that being a responsible patient didn't mean that I had to carry all the responsibility myself.

I thought of a quotation from *Ecclesiasticus*. Lee Sturgeon-Day had mentioned it to me once:

> Hold the physician in honor,
>   for he is essential to you,
> and God it was Who established his profession.
> My son, when you are ill, delay not,
> but pray to God, Who will heal you.
> Then give the doctor his place...
>   for you need him too.
> There are times that give him an advantage,
>   and he too beseeches God
>   that his diagnosis may be correct,
> and his treatment bring about a cure.

I received a very official mailing from Dr. Blasko and Co., requesting all manner of information: records from my physicians, biopsy reports, PSA blood test results, and reports of all x-rays, bone scans, CAT scans, and MRI scans. That was pretty much expected. What impressed me was his request for the original slides of my prostate biopsy. He intended to look at them himself. It was comforting to realize that this physician paid such attention to the details. An accompanying letter from the hospital unbalanced me a bit.

"Although our results are excellent, seed implantation is not an appropriate treatment for everyone. For this reason, we must evaluate your records to make a preliminary decision whether or not you are a candidate for this treatment before asking you to travel to Seattle."

142

I had pinned my hopes on Dr. Blasko and his magic seeds! When I realized that he might turn me down, I again felt that familiar gut ache. I had no backup plan. This had become literally a matter of life and death for me. I was committed to brachytherapy in Seattle.

I shoved my fears down with a little reassuring talk to my internal five-year old, and finished reading the letter. It explained that if I were invited to Seattle, I would be there for a preliminary visit. My evaluation would include yet another study, an ultrasound of my prostate. This ultrasound would be done with a probe in my rectum. (Was there to be no end to things up my rectum?) The ultrasound would accurately measure the size of my prostate gland and allow the physicians to map out the placement of my seeds.

I invited Sherry to accompany me to Seattle. We both knew that this was something we had to do together. I couldn't imagine going through this alone. It was another reminder of how much I value our relationship. I was increasingly depending on Sherry for support.

Knowing that Dr. Blasko would want a current PSA test, I stopped by the lab once again and donated blood to the vampires living among the test tubes and reagent bottles. I was jubilant to find a report on my desk the next morning with a hand written message from the lab. "Congratulations, Doc. Your PSA is less than 0.1! When did you have your prostatectomy?"

I had not dared to imagine that the hormonal therapy

would be so effective. My PSA was so low, the lab could not even measure it! Their most sensitive assay was 0.1. All they could report was that it was "below 0.1"! I'm sure the rumor mill was at work among the vampires. They knew I had prostate cancer and a high PSA just a few months ago. I must have slipped away and had a prostatectomy.

———◦•◦•◦•◦•◦———

On February 10, Sherry and I walked through the doors of The University of Washington's Cancer Center. An hour later I was in the familiar position: on my back, legs spread up in the air with an ultrasound probe up my rectum. I lay in that position with my eyes closed, enduring the indignity for thirty minutes, before I was released and led into an exam room to await Dr. Blasko.

John Blasko, M.D. is a tall, pleasant man with a confident, reassuring air about him. He is soft spoken, and gave us a warm smile when he entered the tiny room. It didn't take me long to know that I was in the right place.

He showed me an inert seed of an iodine isotope. I was struck with its tiny size. I remarked, "It looks like it would fit through an eighteen gauge needle."

"Exactly! Depending on the size of your prostate, we will insert about one hundred such seeds, using as many as twenty-five needles."

I noticed that the thought of twenty-five needles through my crotch didn't seem to bother me very much. I was getting used to the idea. I also knew I would be under anesthesia.

The Doctor soon got down to business. He smiled reassuringly and said, "I've looked over your studies and slides. I'm concerned that the cancer may have already spread beyond your prostate's capsule. Seed implants in your prostate gland won't do the job alone. I recommend combination therapy: a short course of conventional external beam radiation, followed by a two week rest, and then we will do the seed implants."

I wasn't surprised by his recommendations. I had seen this as an evolving pattern. The external beam of x-rays would kill any cancer that had penetrated the capsule of my prostate gland. The radiation dose would be kept low to minimize damage to surrounding organs. Such a low dose could not sufficiently penetrate my prostate gland to kill the cancer. It would be the task of the implanted seeds to sterilize the interior of my prostate.

I told Dr. Blasko, "This will take some coordination with Dr. Rosenthal back home, but I'm sure we can work out the logistics. When do we start?"

"The ultrasound study that we just did shows that your prostate is shrinking rapidly under the effects of your hormonal therapy. If it gets much smaller it will become technically difficult to place the seeds properly. We need to move the timetable up a bit. You should start your external beam therapy as soon as possible, hopefully next week. After that you'll need a couple of weeks to recover before you return here for the seeds. How does April 23rd sound?"

"Great, good things happen on April 23rd! That's

Sherry's birthday."

"OK, you're on the schedule, but first I want to give you some important information about what to expect."

With that introduction, John Blasko reached for a diagram of a man's pelvis and launched into a little talk that I suspect he has given hundreds of times. He explained: "There are several expected side effects of the 'seeding,' which include more frequent urination, feeling of urgency to urinate, and slower urinary stream."

"How long can I expect to experience these effects?"

He reassured me, "Generally, these effects are worst at two-to-six weeks after the procedure; then they slowly decrease until gone—usually by eight to twelve months. We can control most of those symptoms with medications. Unfortunately, one out of ten men develop obstruction of the urethra and require a catheter for one to eight weeks." Oh great, there it is again, the prospect of a catheter in my penis for as much as two months!

Then he added, "I think you will do better with seeds of Palladium 103 rather than the Iodine 125. The Palladium is a hotter isotope. The half life is seventeen days compared to sixty days for Iodine. The total dose will be about the same, it's just delivered faster."

I suspected that with the hotter isotope, Palladium 103, the side effects would arrive swiftly and with more intensity; nevertheless, I liked the idea of using the Palladium. I had seen some concern in the literature, concern that a fast growing cancer might be able to grow and repair itself almost as fast as the radiation of Iodine 125 could kill it.

Dr. Blasko went on to explain that I would be carrying a radioactive source in my pelvis. I should not put small children in my lap, and I should keep pregnant women at arm's length (actually six feet) for about three weeks. He asked that I strain all my urine for a week, in case I expelled a seed. I would be given careful instructions what to do if I found one.

The good doctor then finished by telling me: "There are permanent complications among our patients that I need to tell you about. Three percent of men get an inflamed bladder which manifests as a frequent need to urinate, urgently. Fortunately, incontinence is rare. Two percent of men have had temporary, painless rectal bleeding about one year after seeding. All of these men have healed. None have required surgery. Of all men, 25% completely lose the ability to have an erection. Another 40% find that their erections are less firm than before seeding. The average age of our series is 70 years. Younger men fare better. Do you have any questions so far?"

"Yes; what about convalescence? Should I expect much pain from the procedure itself. Will I feel like going back to work, or should I schedule some off time?"

"Plan to take a week off to convalesce. The only people I send back to work right away are lawyers. These people are used to being a pain in the ass."

Now I knew this was the right man! That's something I might have said.

As we left the clinic I noticed a definite spring in my step. I was sure I had made the right decision. Sherry and I had a few hours to kill before we had to be at the airport. I was feeling adventurous with my new lease on life and hailed a cab. As we entered the back seat, I asked the cabby to take us to a fun place for lunch—his choice. Sherry gave me a look that I knew said: "Why have you just given a total stranger permission to drive us any place he wants, and then charge us for it?" That was OK. I was willing to put my faith in this driver and let him do his job. I would trust in my destiny.

We soon found ourselves in a disheveled neighborhood, entering a small Ethiopian restaurant. The owner came out of the kitchen to greet to us. She was as curious about us as we were about her. Sherry and I had visited Ethiopia as a young couple. We told her that it had been 25 years since we had enjoyed good Ethiopian food. When she heard that, she withdrew to her kitchen, only to reappear with arms full of platters—trays of her best cuisine for our pleasure. It was nectar of the gods! By the end of dinner we had found friendship. She pronounced us her guests and refused to accept payment for our meal!

On the flight home I loosened my belt, giving my stuffed stomach room to digest all that good food. As I rubbed my tummy in satisfaction, I reclined in my seat and pondered life's lessons. I'd learned one about trust that day.

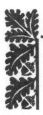

CHAPTER 13

TAKE THAT, YOU SOB'S!

"We'll have to move fast, if you're going to start radiation therapy next Monday."

With those words Dr. Seth Rosenthal launched me onto a whirlwind of preparations for my external beam radiation therapy.

First they had to make a cast of my body. The radiation therapists call it a foam cradle. All measurements and therapy would happen while I was in that cradle. The cradle would ensure that I didn't move during therapy. Through a procedure called **Conformal Beam Therapy**, the radiation would be focused on my pelvis in a narrow beam. That beam would have to be shaped (conformed) like my prostate gland, with about half an inch margin around the perimeter. One half inch—that's all. If the therapist's aim was off, she would irradiate something else in my pelvis—possibly damaging my bladder or rectum, and missing the cancer. So off we went to the cast room.

The therapist asked me to recline on a table with something that felt like a long bean bag under me. Once she had my legs buried in nice bean bag grooves, she attached a hose to the bag and sucked the air out of the bag. Presto, the bag hardened into a comfortable cradle for my legs, and I was immobilized!

"We'll put you into this cradle every time we do measurements or give you therapy." Then she added, "That was the easy part."

"Whatta ya mean: 'easy part,'" I asked. "What's the hard part?"

"Now I have to give you your tattoos."

"Tattoos?"

"No one told you that you would be getting tattoos? They will help us aim the radiation beam."

I saw her reach for a small needle filled with blue ink. I had cared for patients who were undergoing radiation therapy and noticed their small tattoos. Now it was my turn. Once again my internal five-year old started going nuts—ignoring my mature doctor self, who was saying something like: "Shucks, just a few insignificant blue dots where no one should be looking anyway. This is serious stuff, life and death stuff, and we want to get those healing beams on target, don't we?"

My emotional self was aware that I would be marked for life—irrefutable reminders that I had been through prostate cancer and radiation therapy. But somehow it was more than that. I sensed that events had begun to sweep me along into a torrent. I was losing control of events, even though I had set these events in motion. Doors were slamming shut behind me. Choices were fast becoming irreversible.

I recalled the same feeling at my wedding: I was standing at the altar with my best man Jerry. I looked around at smiling faces of friends and loved ones—all the important people in my life—and I was doing just fine. Suddenly the church organ sprang to life, filling the air with the Wedding March. The sound was reverberating against the stained glass windows, so powerful, it was palpable! I looked toward the back of the church and saw Sherry for the first time as my bride. My God, she was beautiful! She was walking to me while holding her father's arm. That's when the reality of what we were doing really struck me. I remember thinking: *"Mike, you are committed now!"*

Of course, commitment is what makes any ritual significant. Rituals create a responsibility for permanence—or change. They produce a sense of demarcation. Anyone going through a significant ritual feels that he or she has crossed a line. These features are found in every wedding, funeral, graduation, Confirmation, and Bar Mitzvah.

Here I was, about to receive my tattoos of radiotherapy. It felt like a meaningful rite was upon me—an initiation into the fraternity of Dr. Roentgen. I resolved to give this moment the importance it deserved. I didn't want to trivialize the event with idle conversation. I gave the technician permission to do whatever she needed and accepted my tattoos in silence.

She put three blue dots on my body—one on each hip and one above my pubic bone. Those three reference points would be used to focus the radiation on my prostate gland during therapy.

"OK, that's it for the day." With a smile she handed

me an instruction sheet.

"Tomorrow you'll have to go to the downtown cancer center. They have a CAT scanner dedicated to cancer therapy. We'll get a CAT scan of your pelvis."

"Will they be looking for spread of the cancer again?"

"No, the purpose is to measure your pelvis. We'll need that information to shape and aim the beam."

"Anything else I need to know?"

"The printed instructions will answer most of your questions. Stop by the drug store and pick up a Fleet's enema. Give yourself an enema before you leave for the center in the morning. You'll need an empty rectum. The technicians will put a catheter in your bladder and rectum. The study is done with contrast material."

Of course! That made sense. X-rays cameras don't see the bladder or rectum well. Contrast material is a dense liquid the cameras can see. The radiologists would use catheters to inject contrast material into my rectum, urethra and bladder. All three organs will virtually light up on the x-ray film. When the radiologists can see the rectum and bladder well, they can shape the radiation beams to avoid damaging those vital structures. I rose from the table with an exaggerated bowlegged gait and headed towards the door. "Thanks for the warning!"

"You're most welcome. We'll see you again next Monday morning to start therapy."

<hr>

The Sutter Cancer Center is a marvel of modern design. I was greeted by a valet at the driveway. Nice touch! The waiting lounge had complimentary coffee and a waterfall under a huge skylight. Interesting how lobbies of hotels and hospitals are beginning to resemble one another. The receptionist greeted me with an awkward smile, "I'm sorry to have to tell you this, but the CAT scanner is tied up doing emergency therapy. Your study had been slipped back an hour." Resigned to my wait, I wandered off to find a seat near the waterfall.

Desperate for something to read, I picked up a stack of pamphlets with advice for cancer patients. One described *The Americans with Disabilities Act*. I read that cancer patients fall under its umbrella. My employer cannot fire me because I have cancer and must make reasonable adjustments to accommodate any handicap I may develop. In fact, it is illegal to consider my cancer during hiring or promotion deliberations. Somehow it was comforting that Uncle Sam was looking out for me. I also knew that no one was going to offer me an emergency department directorship any time soon. My partners knew I would be distracted and going through my own trials for the next year. I was facing probable time off the job and maybe a period of severe disability. This would not be a good time for increased responsibility, regardless of government rules.

———•••••••———

An hour later I was once again semi-naked on an x-ray table. I was pleasantly surprised when the technicians produced my custom-made cradle. Someone had taken the time to drive an hour from Cameron Park and delivered it in downtown Sacramento. This was true commitment to my therapy. The technicians were both attractive young women. I was surprised that I didn't feel the least bit self-conscious about that.

I certainly should have! The first thing they did was insert a catheter into my rectum! I could feel the cool contrast material filling my bowels. They then rolled me onto my back and taped a BB over each of my three tattoos. (The BBs would light up as bright spots on x-ray photos.) Finally the part I had been dreading arrived. One of the women put a catheter into my penis, pushing it up to my bladder. That hurt! She then filled my bladder and urethra with contrast material. As a final indignity, she put a clamp on my penis and turned back towards the control room!

I just spontaneously blurted out, "Hey, this thing is uncomfortable! Are you planning to leave that clamp there on my penis during the entire CAT scan!?"

She looked surprised as she turned back to me, "Really? No one has ever complained about it before."

"You've gotta be kidding! No one has ever complained about a medieval thumb screw on his penis? How long do I have to endure this clamp?"

"The scan takes about fifteen minutes. Think you can stand it?"

"I guess I'll have to."

⊷•●●●●•⊷

For the next fifteen minutes I tried to lie still in my cradle—and ignore the clamp and catheters. Astounding!

No man has ever complained about this clamp before. Was I a wimp? Was the average man so intimidated, that he would endure anything without a peep? I didn't like either possibility.

When the clamp was finally off, I glimpsed at my penis. The poor thing was bruised! Knowing that I had done my share of bellyaching, I ignored the bruise. I thanked the women for their professional care and left for my drive home. In truth, they had done a great job, and it wasn't so bad.

The CAT scanner had produced four views of my prostate gland: front, back, and each side. The BBs prominently showed the radiologists where the tattooed aim points were on my skin. The doctors would mark the films with magic markers, outlining a pattern, which the beam of radiation must follow from each of the four directions. The pattern would include my prostate gland and the tissues extending half an inch around it, with a small bulge to include my vas deferens. The radiation would be routed around my pubic bone, rectum, and bladder. Technicians would then use those patterns to make cast metal ports. The ports would fit over the x-ray outlet and shape the beam. My therapy would start Monday. That meant that the technicians would be busy over the weekend.

———◄●●●●●●●►———

I also had work to do. I had to spend some time on the phone making arrangements for therapy. I cut back my workload and scheduled my treatments in the mornings, Monday through Friday, for the next five weeks. My partners were wonderful. Without complaint they shouldered the extra hours and covered my night shifts.

⸺•••••••⸺

Monday morning arrived soon enough. Sherry volunteered to come with me. I was delighted! I had no idea what my mental state would be, as I lay under that machine for the first time. I knew Sherry's support would be crucial to me.

The radiation technicians greeted us warmly in the lobby. One invited Sherry to watch my therapy. When we entered the therapy room, I was startled by green beams of light crisscrossing the room. It looked like something out of *Star Wars*! As I looked over the lights, I realized that I was almost right. This was *Star Wars!* These were lasers! There was a laser beam coming out of the middle of each of four walls. Another was beaming out of the center of the ceiling. All five beams were intersecting over the center of the treatment table. That's when I noticed my body cradle on the table, glowing green under the lasers. I was to be placed at the intersection of those laser beams! The beam of x-rays would be focused at that green intersection.

Towering over the table was a huge x-ray machine that would generate the invisible beam of radiation. It was designed to pivot about the table, concentrating its lethal beam at the axis of rotation. I knew that the radiologists planned to put my prostate gland at the center of that axis. Here in this surrealistic chamber was the best that modern medicine had to offer. It would be here that I must fight my battle with the killer in my groin.

I don't think anyone had to tell me to get on the table. That was the obvious thing to do. I had to bare my pelvis, and snuggle into the cradle. The technicians maneuvered the motorized table into the laser beams—aligning them with my tattoos. They then rotated the x-ray machine over my body and put a metal port over the "eye" of the machine. That port would shape the beam to fit like a glove over my prostate gland. I was glad to see my name on the port. They had the right one.

I was calm as I lay there at "ground zero." That surprised me a bit. I had already done my worrying. I glanced over to Sherry and was glad she was there for me. As we exchanged smiles, the attendants led her out of the room and turned down the lights.

There I was, alone in this temple of technology. Everyone else had fled the radiation that would soon be flooding the room. A mental image of a sacrificial lamb on the altar flashed through my mind. My nose started to itch. No way to scratch it now. I resisted an urge to turn my head and look for Sherry behind the leaded glass. I was determined to stay exactly as I had been placed on the table. I wanted that beam to be on target! If I squirmed as much as ½ inch, the beam of radiation could miss my prostate gland.

Even though I knew I would feel nothing when the radiation hit me, I had to resist the urge to cringe. I felt a need to lighten up, as I lie there staring up at the x-ray machine. I chose to address the one-eyed Cyclops.

"Take me to your leader, alien!"

It must have heard me! Suddenly it was alive and buzzing.

"This is it!" I said under my breath.

"You're committed now, Doctor Dorso."

"You'd think they would at least play the Wedding March!"

Of course I felt nothing as the machine flooded my pelvis with radiation. I tried to imagine the chaos this was creating in my vitals. I visualized cancer cells looking up in dismay as they began to shrivel, incapable of understanding the forces I had marshaled against them.

"Take that, you Sons of Bitches!"

When the machinery stopped its buzzing, the technicians reappeared, lights on. They rotated the x-ray machine to my right, and changed the metal port to match my prostate's profile from the right. I checked to see that my name was on that one too. Then it was everybody out, lights out, another few seconds of buzzing. We went through this four times: front, back, left, and right.

"Take that, and that, and that!"

And then we were done. The whole process didn't take fifteen minutes. I was dressed and out the door less than thirty minutes after I had arrived. I felt great as Sherry and I walked out into a bright February morning. One down, twenty-four to go.

***

After that, things settled into a routine. I would leave every weekday morning for my therapy and be home again in an hour and a half. I knew I would not need Sherry's support after the first treatment. With time, I befriended several other patients. The camaraderie that developed among us became an ad hoc support group.

The patients' changing room is where it's at! It provided a small waiting area and curtained cubicles where a man or woman could gown for therapy. My first day there I was approached by a woman who recognized me as a physician. She chose to tell me about her illness in great detail. We had a good conversation, while waiting for her therapy. After she left, an attendant approached me with an apologetic tone in her voice.

"Doctor, I'm so sorry that happened!"

"What happened?"

"I'm concerned about your privacy. You looked pretty cornered by that woman. I can arrange for you to wait in a private room, so that won't happen again."

"Oh, God no! Don't stick me in a room alone to stare at four walls. I needed that human contact at least as much as she did."

One day as I arrived at the changing room, I noticed a new patient waiting for therapy. She was an elderly woman with a younger companion—I presume her daughter. I greeted them with a smile and went behind a curtain to undress. As I came out, I was feeling a bit self-conscious in my ravishing hospital gown.

She looked at me and asked, "I'd like to know how many treatments I have to receive, before I'm comfortable enough to come in whistling like that? You look like you're doing well!"

Her comment made me realize that I was doing well. I was in good spirits, and I guess it showed. In fact, I seemed to be doing so well that I felt like a dilettante. There were some patients passing through who were obviously ill—men abnormally thin or vomiting; some in pain; women wearing bandanas over their bald heads. It all sounds pretty grim. It wasn't! These people displayed an amazing spirit. I was repeatedly impressed with the courage they exhibited in the face of such adversity.

One day as I walked across the parking lot after therapy, I noticed a woman retching as she leaned over her car's fender. I walked over to her. She was sweaty, wearing a wig that had slipped askew. I helped her over to the lobby. We sat and talked, as we waited for her physician. She was going through her third round of chemotherapy for breast cancer and would soon start radiation therapy. Between retching, she said, "This chemotherapy is kicking my butt. I sure hope it's worth it!"

And then she smiled! I can only imagine the strength it took to muster that smile.

One evening at work I cared for a forty-two year old woman recently diagnosed with cancer of the anus. She was receiving radiation therapy to her pelvis—eight more treatments to go—and she already had painful burns of her skin. Unable to bear it any longer, she came to the emergency department. When I examined her, I realized that the skin of her pelvis and genitals looked badly burned—an angry red with blisters developing. I couldn't imagine what she would look like after eight more treatments. I had to admit her to the hospital for pain control. I started watching my skin for signs of radiation dermatitis—never found any.

⸺◦◦●●●●●●◦⸺

About halfway through my five weeks of therapy, my body began to rebel. My first symptom was a mild diarrhea. I knew my rectum was becoming inflamed. Seth prescribed Immodium, which stopped the problem. Soon thereafter I developed bladder irritation. I was urinating every twenty minutes and enjoying it less. My bladder was obviously taking a hit in the crossfire of radiation. Taking the anti-inflammatory drug Aleve helped a great deal.

One of the therapists suggested that I arrive for therapy with a full bladder. She advised me, "When your bladder is full, much of it rises out of your pelvis—out of the path of the radiation."

Now each therapy became a balancing act—juggling my morning coffee to arrive with a full bladder, as full as I could stand it. If therapy was delayed fifteen minutes, I was in trouble. My inflamed bladder could become quite insistent. Each session of therapy now ended with a beeline to the bathroom.

———⋯•••••••⋯———

It had become my self-appointed task to check my name on the ports as they were fitted over the outlet of the machine. One day, after therapy, the therapist was helping me off the table. I asked her, "How come all my ports have 'Kowalski' instead of 'Dorso' on them today?"

She just laughed hardily and retorted, "You don't think you're the first patient to try that one on me do you? Next you'll ask me if you will be able to play the piano after your therapy is over!"

———⋯•••••••⋯———

As I was sitting in the changing room one day, a woman I had seen there a few times walked in jubilant. She had just completed her last treatment. She flashed a "diploma" given to her by her therapists. It looked quite impressive. *Of course!* This had to be what my father received with his therapy! He had invested a great deal of hope in that souvenir piece of paper.

———⋯•••••••⋯———

About three weeks into the therapy I began to feel fatigued. I found it tiresome to get through a shift. I wondered if this was depression or the consequence of a dying prostate gland. I found myself taking more naps. Friends began to tell me that I was pale. The lab confirmed that I was developing an anemia. Seth attributed the anemia to the hormone therapy. After about four weeks, I noticed that the hair on my abdomen was disappearing, and my pubic hair was thinning. I suspect that was hormonal too.

By now I had become completely impotent. Somehow it didn't seem to be very important. I had bigger fish to fry, and hopefully it was a temporary condition. Sherry and I settled into a comfortable pattern of physical affection that seemed to meet our needs.

And my therapy settled into a comfortable pattern as well. Mondays I weighed in before therapy. Also on Mondays I received x-ray photos of my pelvis, to verify that the beam was on target. Wednesdays I would meet with Dr. Rosenthal. The therapists were always enthusiastic and attentive. I suspected that I would eventually miss having so much energy focused on my well being.

One day I met a colleague, an urologist, in the hall. I mentioned that I was going through radiation therapy for prostate cancer. When I told him that I intended to fly to Seattle for seed implants, he frowned and said with some alarm in his voice, "You need to talk to me before you start your therapy! Radiation will not give you the long term results that surgery can provide."

I countered, "John Blasko has some impressive statistics."

"Yeah! They're *too* good. Some workers think he is doctoring his numbers, and he has no long term results!"

Realizing that this conversation was going no place good for me, I informed him that the die was cast, and I was half way through my treatment plan. I managed to end the conversation on a cordial note.

Later I had to reassure myself that Dr. Blasko was an

ethical man, and that I had made the right decision. There was no way I would be able to change horses in the middle of this raging river!

———————

As the day of my last treatment approached, I felt a need to celebrate—a closing ritual. My first impulse was to bring champagne to my last day of therapy. Sherry vetoed that. She reminded me that the staff couldn't drink on the job. Instead, I packed a large basket with sparkling cider and wine glasses. I suspected the staff had planned their own ceremony.

Sure enough, after my last treatment, the staff all gathered in the treatment room. They presented me with my "diploma."

"Michael Dorso has completed his prescribed radiation therapy treatments with high honors in courage, cooperation, and good spirits."

I was pleased to see personal notes in the margins by my therapists: Lorraine, May, Carol, Sandy, and Joni.

We opened three bottles of bubbly and drank a toast to my health, to their professionalism, and to modern medicine. After we shook hands, I walked out the door—"cured."

As I think back to that time, I realize that Patty was right. It was a time of purposeful activity, and it felt good. I was kicking my cancer in the ass. It was down, but not yet out.

In two weeks I would be off to Seattle for the final blow.

CHAPTER **14**

SEEDS OF HOPE

"This is a hell of a way to run a business!" The woman next to me was losing it. She was a lovely brunette, a picture of health. I wondered what surgery she was having. We had been sitting in the surgery waiting room for an hour, and nothing seemed to be happening. The University of Washington Cancer Center had called last night and asked us to be there at 7 AM. We arrived at 6:50. We checked in. We sat, worrying.

A second patient, a pleasant looking man, chimed in, "Tell me about it! Could you imagine how long IBM would survive asking clients to show up three hours before their appointments?" I wondered if he too was having seed implants. Then I couldn't resist joining the grousing.

"Not only that, they take your clothes away and won't let you eat after midnight!"

I resisted complaining about last night's meal of soup broth and laxative. My gut was still grumbling about the two enemas I had taken two hours ago. The unspoken complaint that we all shared, of course, was that they also put you to sleep—and then do unspeakable things to you. I was well aware that I would soon receive twenty-two large needles in my crotch!

"Mister Dorso, we're ready for you in pre-op. Can you come with me, please?"

I looked up to see a young man smiling down at me. My heart sank. I hadn't seen him enter the room. Time to go be a real patient. I noticed that he called me *Mister* Dorso. Did anyone around here know I was a physician? I was unsettled by the anonymity that came with being a "mister." Perhaps the truth is that every man with prostate cancer is a "mister"—if the invading cancer bothers with names at all. It is a common denominator, a leveler against every form of status, accomplishment, privilege, or resource.

Sherry and I followed him into pre-op. A large nurses' station lined one wall of the room. A row of curtained cubicles claimed the other side. As I was led to my cubicle, I noticed a diminutive young woman to my right. She was in her hospital robe, with an intravenous line in her left arm. Using less than a third of her chair, she had curled up into a tight ball, her arms wrapped around her flexed knees. Her protective posture and facial tension reminded me of a cornered animal. I wondered what kind of cancer surgery she was to endure. I could see that she would probably welcome sedation. I had to suppress my physician training and remind myself that I was a patient. I wouldn't be ordering any sedation here.

My cubicle was furnished with a large lounge chair that I knew could quickly become a bed in an emergency. I noticed an I.V. pole and wall oxygen. I was greeted by a pleasant nurse who handed me a bathrobe and a blanket, and then asked me to disrobe as she closed the curtain behind her. Sherry and I were alone with only the illusion that privacy curtains provide. I gave her a peck on the cheek. She folded my clothes as I undressed. A close relationship of thirty-four years, at a time like this, was marvelous.

Lying there in my cotton robe, I was undeniably feeling like a patient. Once again the waiting game began. I heard the woman to my right hyperventilate a few times. The nurses moved promptly to reassure her.

My nurse had trouble finding an arm vein for an I.V. I was surprised. In the past I had noticed nice bulging veins in my arms. Where had they gone? Were they hiding? Had my hormone therapy wrapped them in subcutaneous fat?

I was feeling anxiety about the I.V. and told the nurse, "You know, I've never had intravenous therapy before."

"You're kidding! Fifty-five years old and a physician, and you've never had an I.V.?" Then she added, "I could use some local anesthetic if you like."

Great! She knew I was a physician. I wondered if she offered local anesthetic to everyone, or was this VIP treatment? I reassured myself that the answer was obvious. This woman seemed dedicated to her patients, and I was enjoying the same good care that everyone received.

The time dragged, despite visits by the anesthesiologist, Dr. Blasko, and his assisting urologist. I was trying to read the status board across the room; trying to gauge my progress, when I heard the "cornered lady" begin to hyperventilate again. The nurse was with her and attempting once again to calm her.

"You know, you'll be asleep when they do this. You won't feel a thing!"

Cornered Lady was gasping, trying to answer between deep breaths.

"I know, and I've been through this so many times before, but I'm still scared!"

I realized that their voices were fading away. She was being wheeled into surgery! No wonder she was panicking! I heard the reassuring voice of her nurse, sharing her own fears, when she once had surgery. She was doing a wonderful job as their voices left the room. I wished the lady well.

And then it was my turn. A male nurse wearing scrubs walked into my cubicle and asked if I was indeed Dr. Dorso, and then asked, "Would you prefer to walk to surgery? I can push your I.V. pole behind you."

"I would be delighted to walk!" I rose to my feet, kissed my lady for good luck, and headed for the door.

There was something powerful about walking into that surgery suite under my own power. I still haven't figured it out for myself. Perhaps it afforded me some sense of control over events threatening to overwhelm me. There was a sense of dignity in that promenade down the hall. It wouldn't have been the same flat on my back.

I entered an operating room that seemed full of people. They had been waiting and greeted me warmly, as though they were genuinely happy to see me. I half expected everyone to yell, "SURPRISE!" I could see that they had been busy preparing the room. All was in order. The operating theater had a modern warm look with indirect lighting fixtures curving overhead. Gone were walls covered with bathroom tiles that I'd come to expect. Instead the walls were a soft off-white. People were in action all about the room. All scary instruments were discretely in the back, covered with drapes. The operating table had a fresh sheet over its pad.

The charge nurse gave me a friendly smile, asked me to recline on the table, and wrapped me with a warm blanket. That heated blanket was a soothing touch. It felt terrific! Everyone seemed so reassuring! They were obviously focused on my well being.

I felt a mask placed over my face, as the anesthesiologist reassured me, "This is just oxygen. It will help. Expect it to smell a bit like plastic from the tubing." Then he added, "You're going to begin to feel drowsy now, like a good drunk coming on. Don't be alarmed."

I noticed a burn at my I.V., as the drugs flowed into my veins. A few seconds later I felt the mother of all drunks coming upon me. I wondered how long I could remain awake despite the drugs.

My next conscious thought was, "Something is burning fiercely!" It was my penis! I reached down, and felt a catheter protruding from my urethra. That thing had to go!

"Good morning, sleepy head. Will you take a few deep breaths for me?"

Some disembodied voice seemed to be talking to me! I opened my eyes to see my nurse smiling down at me. I was in the recovery room. I'm afraid I wasn't very sociable. I answered her request with a complaint.

"This catheter really hurts for some reason! Can we get rid of it?"

"We usually leave them in until you're fully reactive, but I think we can take it out now."

She removed it with practiced expertise. It was such a relief to shed that tube!

"How long will I stay here?"

"Probably a couple hours. You must be able to walk. It would be good if you kept some food down before you leave. We're in no hurry. You can take all the time you need." Then she asked, "Would you like to see your wife now?"

"No. I'm not ready to see her yet."

I surprised myself with that answer. I just didn't want to have to be nice to anyone. I didn't want to be brave. I didn't want anyone worrying about me and watching my every move—especially the person who loved me more than anyone else in the world. It didn't occur to me that it would have been good for Sherry. She needed to see that I was doing well.

The next couple hours are a blur. I was drifting in and out of sleep. Nurses kept an ice pack in my groin. Somewhere in time, Sherry appeared at my side. I was delighted to have her near me. Eventually I managed to eat a snack and get on my feet. As I was dressing, I realized that my scrotum was twice its normal size, and deep purple! That startled me. I had an ache in my groin, but my scrotum looked like I should be feeling serious pain!

I muttered, "This would be a great opportunity to win some bets in the bar!" Sherry asked with puzzlement, "What did you say, honey?"

"Never mind—just some macho male musings."

Seated on an inflatable doughnut pillow, I said my good-byes to the nursing staff and was wheeled out the door in a wheelchair to a waiting cab.

That evening wasn't too bad. My job was to lie in the hotel bed with an ice bag in my crotch. Pain pills made it tolerable as I watched T.V. I had a constant urge to urinate, and was up frequently trying to pee, but with limited success. Sometime in the middle of the night I passed an obstructing blood clot through my penis—followed by a surge of pent up urine. Now that got my attention! That was probably the most uncomfortable event of the entire therapy. I went back to my bed and drank a quart of water. I wanted thin, dilute urine to wash away any more potential blood clots.

By morning I was on my feet. We were off to the Cancer Center for yet another CAT scan and doctor's appointment. The CAT scan would show exactly where my seeds had been placed. Dr. Blasko had warned me that if he didn't like the placement pattern, he might implant a few more seeds. I chose to ignore that possibility!

The waiting room was crowded. I was keenly aware that I was now radioactive. I pictured photons streaming from my pelvis, like some alien looking for its radioactive mate, to sooth his loins. An obviously pregnant woman sat next to the one available seat. I *knew* I didn't want to sit next to her! I chose to stand alone in a corner. Fortunately it wasn't long before a couple left a double seat empty. I quickly claimed it and was able to curl up on my side. I knew that I was taking up two seats on a crowded day, but I didn't want an unsuspecting patient sitting next to me, in my radioactive state.

John Blasko was pleased with the CAT scan. Thank God! John told me that the hotter seeds were causing more bladder and urethra irritation. Great! I was already having trouble peeing from Dr Rosenthal's Cyclops machinery. I wasn't looking forward to even more symptoms.

Blasko prescribed Cardura to help with my symptoms. As the name implies, Cardura is a **car**diac drug with a long **dur**ation of therapy. It is marketed to treat high blood pressure and works by relaxing the muscle tone in one's arteries. Someone realized that it also relaxes the muscles of the urethral sphincter, prostate, and bladder. A close cousin, Hytrin, has been used for years to relieve symptoms of an enlarged prostate gland.

So, now I had to keep track of four medicines: Cardura, Aleve, Eulexin, and Lupron. We agreed that I would see Dr. Rosenthal every three months and return to Seattle in a year.

The flight home had been a concern for me. I knew I would have trouble sitting for more than a few minutes. My engorged, purple scrotum would not take kindly to coach class airline seats. The pressure on my perineum could just become unbearable. I didn't have much faith in the doughnut pillow.

Fortunately the plane was only one-third booked. I managed to find an empty row of three seats across the aisle from Sherry and reclined the entire flight home. The stewardess was great. Leaving out the details, I told her that I had just been through surgery. She pampered me with pillows, blankets, and juice throughout the flight. Her solicitude confirmed that most people will offer support and human kindness to others, if given the chance.

A few hours later, I was comfortable in my own bed. I remembered that I had to be in Nick's office tomorrow for a Lupron shot. As I nodded off to sleep, I wondered when I would be able to cuddle close to my love without irradiating her. I made a mental note to call Blasko and company A.S.A.P. with that question.

I had a naked dream that night. I suddenly realized that I was standing naked in the middle of a supermarket. Don't ask me what happened to my clothes. Mercifully, the store's power failed—lights out. My relief was short-lived. People began to stare at me in wide-eyed amazement. I could see them just fine. It wasn't so dark in the market after all. More gawking people gathered about me. I looked down to realize that the supermarket was awash in light, radiating from my hugely erect, aching penis!

That was too much! I awoke with a start, feeling more embarrassed than anything else. My genitals were aching. I put a fresh bag of ice in my groin. As Sherry turned out the light, I resisted the urge to look once again at my penis—to see if it was glowing.

As I lay there on the threshold of sleep once again, I said a short prayer of thanks. I had been granted strength to get through it all with dignity. It hadn't been so bad, after all.

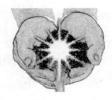

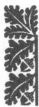

CHAPTER 15

THE ROAD TO RECOVERY

My recovery seemed to go well—for the first week! I actually worked two shifts the next weekend. I was constantly aware that I was carrying a radioactive source in my pelvis, but that seemed more conceptual than real. Sherry and I had thrown all caution to the winds after about a week of sleeping apart. To hell with the radiation! We resumed our usual close sleeping pattern. I quit straining my urine in about three days. To hell with that too! I decided that this low intensity radiation wasn't likely to injure anyone I loved.

Then all hell broke loose! On the night of May Day, I was out of bed every hour to pee. That morning I found myself sitting on the john for thirty minutes with a constant urge to urinate, pondering what was happening to me. I suspected that the radiation was finally making it's presence known. My pelvis was rapidly becoming inflamed.

I called Dr. Blasko's number and spoke once again to Alea. She was concerned that I had developed a urethral stricture and recommended an emergency ultrasound of my bladder to see if it was distended. Fearing the worst, I called Dr. Barnhill. He quickly arranged an ultrasound, and I was on the table in about an hour.

The ultrasound was an uncomfortable experience. I was surprised how tender my pelvis had become, as the technician was probing my lower abdomen—more evidence that the radiation was having its day.

I was relieved to report back to Seattle that my bladder was not distended. I had no serious urethral stricture. My physicians increased the Cardura and Aleve. Dr. Rosenthal prescribed narcotics for relief and recommended that I clear my work schedule for the next two weeks.

My partners were once again terrific. They shouldered about fifty hours of my work without complaint, while I convalesced. Even though I had requested a reduced work schedule before going into therapy, I now realize that I was still too optimistic.

My pelvic irritation calmed down over the next two weeks. While convalescing, I had plenty of time on my hands. I began surfing the net and found a letter by a man who also went through seed implants. He ran half a marathon two weeks after his seeding! There is no way in hell that I could have run anywhere two weeks after my therapy!

———◆◆◆◆◆———

Back on the job two weeks later, I took a dinner break and found myself sitting with the "Coffee Club" once again. One of the physicians greeted me with a smile, "Hey Doc, how ya doing? Is your pecker still glowing in the dark?"

Another grinned and added, "I don't care about that. I

want to know if he's growing tits yet!'"

It seems that male macho behavior and gallows humor are universal phenomena. I accepted their greetings with good humor. I'm sure that's the way it was given. Unfortunately, the second question was striking close to home, as I had noted in my journal the night before. In fact, my journal often stood as witness to the physical limitations I experienced during those months.

<hr>

JOURNAL ENTRY — June 20

It is now seven months since I began my hormone suppression therapy. I had no idea that I would miss my testosterone so much. I've nicknamed this therapy *Reverse Steroids*. This is not just some therapeutic idea that is to be taken lightly. My body is definitely changing. My breasts are enlarging. If this gets any worse, I'll need to try on some training bras!

My energy levels have plummeted. It has become a chore just to walk down the driveway to the mailbox. I've gained about a pound a month. I'm getting fat! Some of my clothing has become unpleasantly tight. Sure, I didn't exercise for a few weeks while recovering from my seed implants, but there's more going on here than my missing two weeks of exercise. I know one cancer patient who took pride in his trim seventy-year old body. He is on the same hormonal therapy and has gained thirty pounds in six months.

JOURNAL ENTRY — June 21

I found myself listening to talk radio recently. They were debating animal rights. The topic was castrating bulls. One caller insisted that castration was cruel to animals. The host explained the practical reasons for removing a bull's testicles: The animal becomes docile, easier to handle, and less dangerous. He also gets fat and lazy. Now when he is butchered, the meat is tender and well marbled with fat. I could relate to all of that. I've been chemically castrated for seven months now, and here I sit—Grade A Prime!

JOURNAL ENTRY — June 22

Three months ago I was walking through a child's playground with Everett. I jumped up, grabbing the horizontal bar—intending to show off a bit. I had done rudimentary work on such a bar in high school gymnastics, and developed a flashy spinning dismount. I was planning a demonstration. Instead, I was aghast when I couldn't get up on the bar! I couldn't even do a chin up.

I have always been proud of my upper body strength—swimming every summer to keep up the muscle tone. It has melted away! I hope I can get it back next year.

I have a large yard that I enjoy maintaining, albeit with the help of a professional gardener, who cuts the grass weekly. Doing hard manual labor in my yard adds balance to my life. Last month I filled a wheelbarrow with wood chips, planning to spread them on a path under the trees. As I pushed the wheelbarrow up the front lawn, I became sweaty and acutely short of breath. I felt pain spread across my chest and could feel my heart pounding. I had to sit in the shade for a few minutes to recover.

I was astounded! A year ago I would have pushed that load uphill without a second thought. I had done it many times. I'm planning a Vermont backpacking trip this fall with my brothers. It's becoming painfully obvious that I will not be carrying a forty-pound pack uphill in this condition!

As a physician, I've been trained to notice subtle physical changes. That same training now makes me painfully aware of changes happening to my own body. My skin has taken on a strange smoothness. In some indescribable manner it feels like a woman's skin. The hair on my abdomen and buttocks is gone! I've lost most of my underarm hair. Fortunately, my beard and scalp hair is stable. My testicles have atrophied. They are now about the size of jelly beans.

Some changes have not been so subtle. It's been at least six months since Sherry and I were able to have sexual intercourse. It's as if the wires from my brain to my penis have been disconnected. Come to think of it, that's exactly what has happened! I embrace my wife, and nothing stirs in my loins. Fortunately, I've had a concomitant loss of libido, so I don't seem to miss the sex too much.

I realized that my libido was depressed
recently when I attended a conference. A
young woman sitting next to me had left the
top buttons of her blouse open. Rather than
being intrigued, I was just annoyed. The
thought struck me, "What is this woman trying
to do by showing her cleavage?" I resisted the
urge to request she button up—definitely out
of character for this red-blooded Italian boy.

JOURNAL ENTRY — June 23

I have one more month of hormone therapy
to go. Do I really want to bare my buttocks to
that needle one more time? I grow weary of
people telling me that I look pale. I knew I was
becoming anemic. It comes with the hormone
suppression. That would certainly contribute
to my abysmal exercise tolerance. It's one
reason I couldn't get the wheelbarrow uphill. I
wonder how fast my hemoglobin levels are
falling. Am I becoming dangerously anemic?

I decided to discuss my options with Dr. Seth
Rosenthal. He was gracious enough to see me on short
notice—the day before my last shot of Lupron was due.
Seth and I both know that eight months of hormone
therapy is somewhat arbitrary. The ideal duration of
therapy probably lies somewhere between two months
and two years. I told him that I really didn't want to take
that last shot of Lupron, and that I wanted to stop the
Eulexin.

One thing I'll say about Seth Rosenthal. He is blunt.

"I'm not going to collude with you against Dr. Blasko.

I suggest you call him and see if he has strong feelings about your remaining on the medications. See if he can talk you into hanging in there one more month."

Then Seth added, "Most of the local physicians prescribe four months of therapy. There is a study going on in Canada where patients are taking the medications for two years. We'll eventually see how they do."

That afternoon I called Dr. Blasko's office and spoke to Alea. She advised me, "The Doctor is in surgery, but I'll be glad to convey your concerns to him and have him return your call."

As I hung up, I realized that I didn't want Dr. Blasko to call back. I needed to know that I had done everything possible to defeat this cancer. I didn't want to hear myself one day saying, "If only I had taken the full course of therapy, I may have been cured."

I called Alea again and canceled my request. The next day I drove to Dr. Simopoulos' office for my last Lupron injection.

The story of Saul's conversion on the road to Damascus has always contained an enigma for me. The fact that God was once so willing to directly communicate with a man is comforting. What is puzzling is that it does not seem to happen in modern times. Maybe we just aren't listening. On the other hand, I'm not so sure Saul was listening either!

Instead, I have assumed that God sees a need to distance Himself a bit. That frees us to stew in our own juices awhile and to make our own choices. Let's face it; there can't be much of a free choice for good or evil, if God intervenes every time we stray from the right path. I have always looked askance at some of the more prominent ministers who claim to receive revelations from God.

I tried mightily as a youth to communicate with God; however it all seemed like one way traffic. I listened! I was attentive at the listening post, but I heard no incoming messages. I may as well have attempted extraterrestrial communication. I later realized that God's answers were far more subtle—often appearing as good fortune, or unexpected help from a friend, or possibly advice from a teacher. Hearing the voice of God was not going to happen for me. No, there would be no light permeating the room, no booming voice from heaven.

But something happened on a Sunday that June. I heard Him! I've actually been reluctant to talk about it, for fear of being declared delusional. On the other hand, I've exposed so much of my soul, I may as well let it all hang out.

I was in church, trying to stay awake that morning, and went to the altar for communion. In truth, my mind was wandering that day. I was having trouble staying with the service. If ever I was asleep at the listening post, this was it. Everett was one of the priests at the altar. I had received the host from Rev. Lewis. Everett brought the chalice of wine to me. As he turned away, I was suddenly aglow with an emotional warmth. It was definitely an emotional rather than physical sensation. It was so powerful, that it threatened to overwhelm me. As I stood at that altar, a sense of well being seemed to permeate to my core. No, I didn't hear any voices, but somehow at that moment, I knew I was cured! I still carry that conviction.

I've tried to share this story with friends and colleagues a few times. Typically, their eyes glaze over; they start looking uncomfortable; and I lose eye contact. I began to sense that I was embarrassing them and myself. I've given up trying to tell that story. I wonder how many other people have given up trying.

On July 25, one month after my last Lupron injection, I stopped the Eulexin. I was no longer on hormone suppression. Finally! I invited friends over for a hormone party, just a small gathering of intimate friends. Time to celebrate a milestone on my way back to health. I know how important fellowship can be to us all—especially in times of illness and recovery. There's something intangible that passes between caring people that sustains us. I'm reminded of nurseries in early orphanages, where babies would die, if not handled frequently.

For the party, I challenged all revelers to dress in their best impersonation of a hormone. My offspring began to suspect that we'd gone off the edge of sanity. We toasted my return to health. It was good to be surrounded by friends. I declared myself cured that night. That was emotionally important for me and my friends.

A week later I cared for yet another patient with prostate cancer. Nick Simopoulos referred him to the emergency room for urgent evaluation. The poor man was dying! He had been through a radical prostatectomy years ago. The cancer recurred, and now he was terribly ill. He was dramatically anemic because the cancer was destroying his bone marrow's ability to produce red blood cells. His bladder was over-filled with urine. I suspect the cancer had obstructed his urethra. He was in a great deal of pain with cancer in his spine.

I admit that I was shaken by the experience. My conviction that I was cured was certainly shaken! I remember thinking, "Damn, this is a bad disease! It really can kill me!" I stabilized his condition and arranged for his hospitalization under Nick's care.

Nick called me after work that night. Nick and I have enjoyed a good professional relationship, but he has never called my home. I was truly touched. He knew that I would be disturbed by my encounter with his patient. He literally apologized. I thanked him for his concern and told him that an occasional reality check was good for me.

Later, I pondered my good fortune in having such fine colleagues for physicians. Nick had done a masterful job of guiding me to the right therapy—for me. His patience had rivaled that of Job. He was the one who first mentioned brachytherapy. He never showed disappointment in the path I chose, and supported me whenever possible. Nick certainly refutes the image of a knife happy urologist.

I owe my life to Bradley Barnhill who found the cancer in the first place. A thorough, competent physician, what a blessing!

Seth Rosenthal was a wellspring of information and support. He is truly an authority in the field of radiation therapy for prostate cancer. I value his honest, blunt, no-frills bedside manner.

One morning in mid-September I awoke with an erection. I have no idea why it appeared that morning. I don't remember any erotic dream. I was delighted, but it was another three weeks before another one appeared.

On September 24th I tested my PSA for the first time since my seeding. I was delighted to hear that it was again less than 0.1. My blood hemoglobin was rising, and my stamina was returning. Everett and I hiked back up to Carson Pass for old times' sake. The uphill trails were tough going for me, but I made it! Everett was patient with me on the slow hard climbs. In all, it was a great day. I came home that night to a candle light dinner. Sherry had prepared it, in celebration of my return to Carson Pass.

I visited Seth Rosenthal three days later. He told me he could no longer feel the nodule on my prostate. I did not know he had ever felt a nodule! Seth congratulated me when he saw my minuscule PSA value. Then he warned me, "Your PSA is still being suppressed by the Lupron as well as your radiation therapy. Now that you're no longer taking Lupron, your PSA may rise a bit. Don't let yourself panic with your next PSA testing."

We discussed my inability to generate a good erection. He counseled: "Give it more time. The Lupron has a long-term effect. You will be feeling its influences through Christmas. It's too early to discuss impotence. We don't really know if you have a problem or not." He paused for a moment and added, "My patients seem to have the best results with injections, once they get past the squeamishness of sticking a needle in their penis."

Despite all my reading, I had no inkling that Lupron was so persistent. That really meant that I would be hormone suppressed for about a year in all. I hoped my body still knew how to manufacture male hormones. I was also getting used to the idea of injecting medications into my penis—if that's what it came to. I was content to let the matter lie for a while longer.

———————

I know one co-worker at the hospital who also has prostate cancer. We are of comparable age and were diagnosed at similar stages of cancer. He elected to go to Loma Linda Medical Center for proton beam therapy. He towed his RV there and stayed for about two months. For therapy he received twenty-five treatments with conventional external beam radiation therapy—much like I received. The Loma Linda physicians then gave him fifteen treatments with the proton beam. Basically he substituted a proton boost to his prostate for the seeds I chose. He also elected to avoid hormonal therapy. He tells me that he is doing well. He had such a good time with his RV experience, that he was considering retiring, and living full time on the road.

One day while sharing lunch, he told me that his PSA had fallen to three. His physicians reassured him that three was a good number at this stage, and he could anticipate that it would continue to fall. The prostate cells take a while to die off. I avoided any discussion of my PSA. It would have served no useful purpose to tell him that mine was less than 0.1.

By October, I was well into writing this book. Back in May, I had visited the *WellnessWeb* on the Internet and found the posting by Bart Moran in which he made an eloquent argument for watchful waiting. (You've seen some of his thoughts in chapter ten.)

I sent e-mail to Bart, requesting permission to quote his work. I was shocked to find a return message the next day:

"Unfortunately our beloved founder, Bart Moran, died of complications of prostate cancer on October 1. The rest of us, still in shock, are attempting to bring WellnessWeb along and make it better than ever as a tribute to this great man."

Died! My God, how did this happen! The news brought back that familiar ache in my gut. His numbers were so similar to mine. This could have been me! How did this "champion slow grower" malignancy become suddenly so deadly?

———◄●●●●●●●●►———

I don't know what caused Bart's untimely death. I can't help but wonder: would this dynamic man still be alive if he had elected more conventional therapy? However, it would be unfair to use the irony of this man's death to discredit watchful waiting. I'm convinced that there is merit to those ideas he championed. I felt a great sense of loss for this man I never knew! Another soldier down on the battlefield of cancer. When were we going to get a handle on this killer?

I promised myself I would stay involved with WellnessWeb[1] after writing my book.

[1] WellnessWeb can be reached on the Internet at http://www.wellweb.com

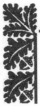

CHAPTER 16

THROUGH THE DRAGON'S BELLY

Like a character in a fairy tale,
one weaves one's way
through a maze of trials
and enlightenments.
One minute one is in the stench-filled
belly of one's dragon-self,
and the next, one is on the mountain top.
The way out of the dragon's belly
is rarely exhilarating,
but the struggle can be magnificent
—in retrospect.

Margaret Gorman

Margaret Gorman is an eloquent friend of mine. I was moved by her images of life's trials—so much so, that I almost chose her image as this book's title.

Going through the stench-filled belly of a dragon seems to describe what I've endured over the last year. It has changed who I am. I'm not the same person as the one standing at a Carson Pass cave a year ago. It is not an obvious change. Instead, it's a transformation in attitude. I have reordered my priorities—what deserves my attention and concern. I don't seem to sweat the small stuff as much.

I'm also getting better about the big stuff! I sometimes stop to realize what I have done. *I have put ninety-*

two radioactive seeds in my prostate gland and allowed them to burn out while embedded in my groin. Who knows what consequences that will have over my remaining years? As a physicist and physician, I've learned to respect the power inherent in any radioactive source. I could spend my creative energies in torment over the long-term effects of that radiation. My bladder and rectum have been seriously irradiated. Am I to deal with bladder or rectal cancer some day?

I could also consume my remaining time left on this Earth in concern over a resurgent prostate cancer.

One takes wisdom from wherever it arises. I'm reminded of a movie I saw many years ago. I'm not sure I even saw much of it. It involved the improbable combination of a kung fu master in a wild west movie. In the scene I remember the Master is sleeping in a slow moving wagon, on top of the cargo. Thugs are somewhere behind—in hot pursuit—on fast horses.

One exasperated character wakes the Master and asks, "Aren't you worried? Those bad guys are going to catch us!"

I will never forget the master's reply: "If I worry, will it make us go any faster?"

That's a lesson I have learned. If worry is futile, why allow it to consume my energies? The future really will take care of itself.

In reflecting back on the past year, I realize that it was a busy, dynamic year. Nowhere in my story did I mention that I was bored. *I continued living my life.* I worked a reasonably full schedule, found time to get out under the stars with friends and telescopes, managed to get through a law suit, corresponded daily with my son at the University of Cairo, cheered for my daughter on the basketball court, went through my mother's funeral, cared for a yard full of roses, found time for medical studies, made love, enjoyed my grandchildren, hosted a Christmas Eve open house, and hiked along the beach. It was a hell of a ride.

Life doesn't end when you have cancer. Instead, it becomes vastly more precious. I find myself reluctant to waste any cherished moment. I will no longer vegetate in front of the TV, as I have in the past. I'm less willing to spend any precious time in anger, argument, long committee meetings, or unnecessary trips.

There have been enlightened views from the mountaintops, as well. I actually feel in partnership with my God. That partnership demands a confidence in His intentions to make this life meaningful—intentions to give me what I need, not necessarily want. There's no guarantee that all lessons will be pleasant, nor all lesson plans obvious. Some lessons can only be learned the hard way.

I can now see my struggle for what it was: an opportunity for my soul's growth. It's another opportunity to "weave one's way through trials and enlightenments" of life. Hopefully, I can be more philosophical when the next illness arrives; and I can be sure it will—sooner or later. I'm willing to trust my destiny.

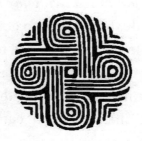

I have accepted my mortality. At first blush, that sounds depressing. I submit that it can be liberating! I have grasped the opportunity in my work, to speak to those who have experienced "near death." These are people who have been gravely injured and have returned to the land of the living. I've met more than one person who described floating near the ceiling—watching us work on his or her body. One woman remembers moving towards a bright light. The stories go on and could make an interesting book some day.

The common theme that permeates their stories is the feeling of peace within themselves. Death no longer holds much fear for them. They no longer spend their energies agonizing over their eventual demise.

I especially remember one man who almost died of a heart attack. I had to shock his heart to revive him. (As we say in the E.R., "He was living better electrically.") In private conversations at his bedside, he told me of his out-of-body experiences. He insisted that he was no longer afraid to die.

A year later he suffered a second heart attack and returned by ambulance. He did well. When I was sure he would recover, I asked him, "How did you feel about the danger you were under? Were you concerned that you might die?"

Without pause he answered, "Doc, I'm not afraid of dying, and you'll never understand how good that feels, unless you experience it yourself." Then he smiled and added, "but I'm not quite ready to go yet!"

———◦•●●●●●◦———

Living life as an asexual being has been instructional, to say the least. Actually, "asexual" isn't really the right word. Sherry and I have continued to be sexual, but sexual intercourse as we used to know it has been denied us. I've come to realize how important the other aspects of intimacy can be. I've learned that making love does not have to equal sex; furthermore having sex does not have to equal intercourse.

Sherry and I knew that once. We rediscovered that truth "in the stench-filled" dragon's belly. Once we comprehended this truth, we were able to relax and rediscover our bodies. I've developed a loving appreciation of my wife and found what strength there can be between two people committed to overcoming adversity. I've learned to express the softer side of myself as a loving mate.

———◦•●●●●●◦———

What advice do I have to offer?

KNOW YOUR PSA NUMBER. DON'T PANIC!

This quick and easy blood test for cancer is a revolutionary concept! There have been other such tests in the past for various malignancies, but never anything this good. You can be sure that there will be more to come. Can you imagine how it would revolutionize the treatment of breast cancer if such a blood test existed? The literature is already talking about refinements of the PSA.

If you are ever diagnosed with prostate cancer, don't panic! Easy to say. Near impossible to do. Remember that this cancer is a champion slow grower. You could reasonably hope for another ten years if you did nothing.

EDUCATE YOURSELF.

You have time to think about options, to talk to survivors. I took too much time. I stalled too long (over six months!) while dealing with my obvious denial and fears. Seth Rosenthal's advice was the best, "Give yourself a month to make your decision, but then you'll need to move on this." He got me off the dime and gave me an objective.

GET A COMPUTER, AND LEARN HOW TO USE IT.

There's a wealth of information and support on the Internet. One outstanding web site is called *Prostate*

Pointers (http://www.prostatepointers.org), maintained by Gary Huckabay. Gary is now in his mid-fifties and was diagnosed with prostate cancer at age forty-eight. He has a wife, two children, and a Ph.D. in mathematics. He tells me, "After my diagnosis and subsequent treatment, the general lack of general information about intelligent treatment decisions became a major bone in my throat." Gary is obviously computer literate and has made it a life's work to maintain this amazing web site. He will refer you to so many places from Prostate Pointers that the possibilities become endless.

It was on *Prostate Pointers* that I found an email support group called *"The Circle,"* which can be found via the Internet at http://www.prostatepointers.org/circle. *The Circle* is made up of men with prostate cancer and their families. They can be a source of information, counsel, and strength. I recently read a posting by an anguished woman. Her husband found out he had prostate cancer as they were planning their honeymoon!

I once printed out an eight-page *Prostate Cancer Resource List* posted by Julie Freestone at this site. Many resources, books, more web sites, and phone numbers of mainstream organizations such as The American Cancer Society can be found at http://prostatepointers.org/prostate.

I retrieved twenty-three pages of dietary advice from what is known as the CaP Cure Nutrition Symposium. (http://www.capcure.org). CaP Cure is a foundation committed to finding a cure for prostate cancer and full of information. It was founded by Michael Milken after he discovered he had prostate cancer at the age of forty-eight.

I recently became aware of the expanded website of http://www.cooleyville.com/cancer, faithfully updated by Don Cooley since his diagnosis in 1997. He has been a proponent of seed treatment. I've included information about Don's website in the appendix of this book.

One last web site I can recommend is PSA-Rising (http://psa-rising.com). This is an on-line news magazine that tracks the latest developments in therapy and activist activity. It can link you with multiple other web sites. You will find encouraging letters and support there.

The National Cancer Institute has a number I'll never forget (1-800-4-Cancer), which will put you in touch with The Cancer Information Service.

 READ! READ EVERYTHING YOU CAN FIND!

Any major bookstore seems to have a half dozen books about prostate cancer. Some of them are unbelievably clinical and boring—a few are excellent.

One good one is *Man to Man, Surviving Prostate Cancer* by Michael Korda (Random House ISBN: 0-679-44844-6). Michael underwent radical prostatectomy for his therapy. It's the first book I read after I learned that I had cancer. I strongly recommend it, especially for anyone considering surgery.

Aubrey Pilgrim has written a laudable book, *A Revolutionary Approach to Prostate Cancer* (Sterling House ISBN: 1-156315-0867). It's the most complete I've seen, without being a textbook. Aubrey is a retired chiropractor who writes in an easy style. He underwent a prostatectomy himself in 1992. He includes a worthwhile chapter of resources at the back of his book. The list is extensive. It includes support groups, journals, newsletters, organizations, and Internet addresses—more leads than you could ever follow. You can order it from him over the Internet: Apilgrm@aol.com. The proceeds from his book go to Patient Advocates for Advanced Cancer Treatments.

Don Kaltenbach is a prostate cancer survivor who has written *Prostate Cancer, a Survivor's Guide* (Seneca House Press ISBN: 0-9640088-2-3). He had palladium seeds implanted in his prostate gland. He goes into detail about the procedure and his recovery. His book features an appendix, "Where to get help" with even more leads to follow.

———•••••••———

If you would prefer a video presentation, I can recommend a fifty-two minute video by Tracy Moore, *Help Yourself*. Tracy was diagnosed with advanced prostate cancer at age fifty-two. He's still out there—thriving. In his video he gives an optimistic message. The video lists resources available to any man with prostate cancer. Call (318) 325-2625 to order the tape. Proceeds support ongoing plant medicinals research through XyloMed Research Inc.

SPEAK TO PHYSICIANS ACROSS THE SPECTRUM OF SPECIALTIES.

As a minimum, I would talk to a urologist and a radiation oncologist. If you are concerned that both types of doctors have a bias towards their own specialty, you can see an oncologist. I did that and greatly valued his unbiased advice. Anticipate that you may get conflicting advice. Much of medicine remains an inexact science.

REMEMBER YOUR LADY.

She will need your support! It is too easy to become self absorbed at a time like this. I guarantee that your mate will be profoundly stressed. Stop to think about this for a minute. She is suddenly faced with the prospect of losing her loved one. Not to mention the possibilities of nursing her man through a prolonged illness, to find herself alone in the world. Then of course she's concerned about lost sexuality, financial ruin, and a myriad of other imagined or real possibilities.

Society will cast her in an impossible role. She is expected to be strong, supportive, loving—all the while never looking sad or needing support for herself. You will need to find the inner strength to deal with her fears, as well as your own.

This, of course, applies to all partners, be they female or male. Anyone committed to you will face the challenge: to find the inner strength for whatever the future holds. If you are living alone, without a partner, I urge you to reach out to family and friends. This is not a time to go it alone.

Julie Freestone has said it so eloquently in her poem:

What If

In the gray, cold night
is when I come face to face with fright.
What if there are no answers?
What if there is no cure?
What if we don't read that one important study?
What if there is no next year?
What if the choice we made is wrong?
And what If I grow old without you here?
That is my repeating, midnight song.

Include your lady in your therapeutic decisions and care. Take her to the doctor with you. Getting her involved will give her perspective and allow her to talk to your healers. She will need a chance to ask her questions as well. Expose her to the light of knowledge. It will dispel the darkness of fear.

 TALK TO HER!

If there is ever a time when you will need clear communication, this is it! The silent, male model doesn't work here. A woman always wants to know what is going on in her man's heart and soul. This especially resonates in times of crisis. Don't be afraid to discuss your fears. Share your concerns over money, disability, impotence, pain, physical deformities, dependence, whatever. If she knows you at all, she will know when you are upset, but she can't read your mind. You need to frame the picture for her.

I know one man whom I diagnosed with chronic leukemia—another champion slow growing cancer. In the best macho tradition, he carried that diagnosis alone for two months. He didn't want to upset his wife. He asked me to be present when he finally broke the news to her. When she heard the diagnosis, she shocked me with her response. With a great sigh of relief she exclaimed, "Is that all? Thank God! I thought you didn't love me anymore!"

 ## TALK ABOUT YOUR SEXUALITY— TO YOUR PARTNER.

Men seem to have more trouble than women talking about their intimate feelings and erotic needs. You will have to overcome your chauvinistic leanings. It seems to be one of life's paradoxes, that sometimes a frank sexual discussion can be most difficult with the one sharing our bed! Bizarre isn't it? You may have looked into her eyes as you shared thousands of orgasms; and yet find it difficult to look into her eyes and discuss your new sexual concerns.

Believe it or not, it can be worse for lovers in long-term relationships. If you're involved in a relationship for decades, you've set down patterns of behavior and communication that will persist, despite how much you've both changed over the years. Many sophisticated middle-

aged couples are still operating under ground rules estab-
lished as teenagers—possibly virginal teenagers. By age
fifty those patterns can become etched in stone.

Men feel especially vulnerable when discussing their
fears of impotence. This is big time body image stuff!
Ignoring this subject won't work. That's somewhat akin to
ignoring a two-ton rhinoceros in the room. Impotence will
not be ignored. Opening a conversation about your apprehensions could be a liberating experience.

Remember that by the time many women reach our
age, they are much less concerned about appearance and
sex than you imagine. Your mate's prime concerns will be
your welfare, your state of mental health, your happiness.
Touching, cuddling, being held are all an integral part
of love making for a woman—much more so than for
men. As women mature, these expressions of love
become even more important. Men are more goal-ori-
ented towards vaginal penetration and orgasm.

Don't let fears of sexual failure stand between you
and the woman you love. You don't have to be a sexual
machine to hold your woman's interest and love. Take
comfort in this. You may be surprised to discover how she
responds to the romantic, intimate, gentler aspects of your
manhood. You may find her eager to have this conversation. She will probably be willing to try some of the erection aids available, should that become necessary.

EXPECT DEPRESSION.

It will affect both of you. It may be subtle, presenting as a lack of energy, a loss of sexual interest, sleeping more, or losing weight. One way out of this deep well is through honestly sharing your feelings. Acknowledging your depression to yourself and your spouse is the first critical step in dealing with these feelings. Intimacy is all about honesty and vulnerability.

Honesty means more than telling the truth. It means behaving honestly. It's permissible to look depressed, when you are depressed. Acting cheerful, when it's not in your heart, seldom comes across as genuine. You'll never be able to fool a woman who loves you anyway! Let her into your heart. Discuss your fears, anger, sense of loss. When you find the strength to come out of this together, you will energize those bonds of love you've forged over the years.

Remind yourself that you are not thinking clearly when depressed. It's easy to attribute ulterior motives to people's best intentions. It's easy to dwell on the negative. It's easy "to cop an attitude." I'm reminded of a successful series of ads for a premium whiskey. The ad simply shows their distinctive bottle half-filled with liquor and asks the question, "Is the bottle half full or half empty?"

Both views are correct of course, but what you see speaks volumes about your approach to life. The optimist sees a bottle still half filled. Plenty of liquor left. No need to worry. The pessimist can become gravely concerned that half of the liquor is missing! The paranoid can muse over who drank all that whiskey. Regardless of what you think, it's the same bottle. It doesn't give a damn how you feel about it! It just is. You get to choose whether to worry about it, or to take comfort from it.

You also get to take comfort from the fact that most men do not die of their prostate cancer; or you can agonize over the thirty-some thousand men who succumb yearly to their disease.

 ### DON'T ALLOW YOURSELF TO BECOME ISOLATED.

It's peculiar how alone a man can feel at a time like this. Some of this isolation is self-generated from within. It's easy to feel set apart. I remember listening to friends planning their retirements. Fearful that I might not make it to retirement age, I found it difficult to join the conversation. Conversations about 401-K investments can seem trivial, contrasted to one's struggle for personal survival. That altered perspective can set you apart. Resist that tendency for all you're worth.

Friends can feel awkward around you. Some may disappear. That's easy to understand. You are a reminder of their own mortality. Our society places premiums on youth, health, and sexuality. We don't deal well with illness, disability, or death. We're unpracticed in the social etiquette of illness. What does one say to a man with newly diagnosed cancer? "So, how's the cancer doing?" It's up to you to break the ice.

This is a time when friends and family will rally around you, if you give them the chance. They will naturally want to support you in your time of crisis. If you seem comfortable with your illness, they will be comfortable discussing it with you. Seek them out. Create the time and structures for them to be there for you. Remind yourself that it is good for a person to contribute to another.

It's OK to be a little selfish at this time in your life. You may find that you are limited in what you can do by your cancer. It's OK to ask for help.

 DON'T MAKE ANY RASH DECISIONS.

This is good advice to follow through any crisis. Hold a steady course at least until you can really see where this cancer is going to take you. Avoid any major life changes, such as quitting your job, moving to that retirement subdivision, divorcing, adopting, remodeling, or any number of other changes that will require you to adapt. Cutting back on your work or other commitments is not a bad idea, if you can do that gracefully.

You will find that being diagnosed with a potentially lethal disease will bring tension enough into your life. You don't need to go out and manufacture any other stressors. This is not a good time to buy a new home or change jobs. This is definitely no time to take on a new lover—or new car payments. The down payment for either seem bad, but the upkeep can be a killer.

CONSIDER SEEKING OUT A CANCER SUPPORT GROUP.

I found mine on the Internet. Perhaps I should say that another found me. I stayed in contact with many of the men who called me for advice and conversation. We formed an informal telephone grouping that was a Godsend. Even though I never met many of these men face-to-face, I consider them friends.

Every town of any size has support groups for all manner of cancer. Contact your local office of The American Cancer Society. The Internet lists every city in North America with a support group—down to the phone numbers of contact persons at: http://www.prostate-pointers.org/prostate/pcsup.html. Just click onto "Support Groups" when the menu appears.

CONSIDER STARTING HORMONAL THERAPY EARLY.

It will stop the clock. You'll have time to breathe. As I review my care, that is one thing I would have done differently. I would have been on Lupron months earlier. Don't let that PSA creep up on you! Your PSA remains the single most important number in this illness. If you have the chance, do whatever you must to keep it below fifteen—preferably below ten.

Of course, there are many who would disagree with that advice. There are as many opinions on treating this disease as there are doctors. Some people consider the side effects of hormonal therapy unacceptable. I consider dying of metastatic cancer unacceptable! I endured hormonal therapy for most of a year. It wasn't that bad. Others may tell you that hormonal therapy should be reserved as an ace in the hole—to be used if all else fails. Well, that's another approach. I chose to follow the advice of Andy Grove and Dr. John Blasko. I gave it my best shot right up front.

 CELEBRATE!

Give recognition to every skirmish won, every milestone passed. It will give you a sense of movement. I toasted the end of my therapy. I celebrated my return to Carson Pass. Save a cigar for the first time you successfully make love after your therapy. Drink champagne when the PSA falls. Reward yourself with a day off for being a good patient. Even if it's a candy bar after your last rectal exam, it's emotionally important.

 DON'T FORGET YOUR FAMILY.

Most of us no longer have small children in the household, unless they're grandchildren. My six-year old grandson is in our home. Like most small children, he can be deeply intuitive. He knew something was going on. I realized that I needed to give him some frame of reference—hopefully with some optimism. I decided to directly address the diagnosis.

"Jordan, Grandpa has a tiny cancer in his belly. I'll have to have some treatments, but I expect to be cured."

I knew I needed to say this with conviction. Jordan would respond to the emotional undercurrent carried in my message. I must have succeeded. He seemed satisfied with my explanation.

My children are all adults or near adults, and I treated them as such. They were a source of strength for me. Involve them early in your diagnosis.

My parents weren't willing to deal with my illness. I realized, somewhat belatedly, that it's difficult for parents to deal with their child's cancer, regardless of their child's age. They also want to hear that you have a little problem, but it's under control.

My mother died—of cancer no less—just before I began my radiation therapy. I flew home to join my family for the funeral. Alone that night in my old room, I noticed a photograph Mother had framed and placed on the dresser. I was repeatedly drawn back to that haunting photo and made this journal entry:

"Last night in my room, I found a photo of myself, age seven, with the ever present fever blister on my lower lip, blond hair, my mother's eyes, shoulder straps on my shorts, nicely pressed shirt with collar—an innocent child staring at me across fifty years of life. I know that child was impatient to become an adult. I remember thinking, 'This is taking so long! Will I never grow up?'"

I found myself looking back across the gulf between us—now as a father of four children of my own, a grandfather with prostate cancer, a physician, husband, lover, church elder, mature human being—wanting so much to communicate with that child looking at me.

Here I am now, contemplating my own mortality at the hands of a cancer in my groin. Hell! That child didn't even know he had a prostate gland!

I looked at that small child's smooth skin, and wished someone had really gotten my attention, and warned me about sun exposure. Ditto brushing, flossing, and cavities.

There is so much I would like to say to this child! I would tell him that he has fifty exciting years ahead—maybe many more. I would tell him: Don't sweat the small stuff. Relax. Have faith in your destiny."

I would now add some other reassurances to that advice: Your soul mate has arrived. She is alive and well in Louisiana. Be patient. You'll get to meet her in about thirteen years.

I would say: Cancer will touch the lives of those close to you and will eventually enter your life as well. There will be times when you will doubt your value, your faith, your future, and your own stamina. You need not fear. You will be given the means to overcome even these doubts.

And finally: Yes, you truly are special! Give yourself

a lifetime to understand this truth.

I open my heart and mind
to the Spirit Rays
of Healing and Knowing.
So that in each moment of life
I experience Joy and Peace.
Endless possibilities exist
for Thinking, Feeling, and Willing.
I live what is Right.
I know what is True.
My life extends beyond purpose.
I share Wisdom with others.

A Healing Meditation
Rosemary Wakeford-Evans

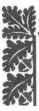

CHAPTER 17

A TIME TO HEAL

To everything there is a season,
and a time for every purpose under heaven:
A time to be born,
And a time to die;
A time to plant,
And a time to sow;
A time to kill,
And a time to heal…

Ecclesiastes

Time sure *does* fly when you're having fun. It's hard to realize that it has been three years since my therapy. Three years of healing. Three more years of life, borne by this fifty-eight year old frame. I wish I could say that a great deal has happened. Truth is, life has been reasonably smooth. I'm actually ecstatic to report that fact.

I've recovered from the therapeutic insults inflicted upon my body with surprising resilience. I've continued to work a full load in a frenetic emergency department and held up well. My strength is back. I finally went on a diet last year and shed the ten pounds I gained while on hormonal blockade therapy. The hair has returned to my chest, abdomen, and underarms. My anemia is gone.

Eleven months after my seeding, I posted this memo to friends on The Circle:

Yesterday was a watershed for me, and I wanted to share it with you. I went snow-shoeing in the Sierra Mountains. Thanks to El Nino, there was ten feet of snow everywhere. The scenery was breathtaking. I went alone, because I wanted to be alone with my thoughts and my God. What better place than His cathedral?

I also went alone because it was my first time out in almost two years! I lost a year with my therapy. Frankly I had doubts that I would be able to keep up with any friend I invited along. It's been a slow recovery from almost a year of "chemical castration." (I still hate that term.)

I did well, my strength fast returning. An hour into my hike, I found myself standing on a ridge, looking down a thousand feet at the Lake Tahoe Basin. *God it felt good!* I felt depression washing away, a quiet depression that I've borne for eighteen months.

As I stood there enjoying the moment, I wondered out loud, "How many years do I have left to do this? Is the beast in my loins really gone, or just subdued?"

Cancer has given me a new perspective on life. I've had to face the possibility that life could be over soon—which is true for any human being. Any one of us could be run over by a Mack truck in the morning. It's just a bit different when the Grim Reaper gets in your face!

This sense of my own mortality has made life evermore precious. I've taken a concept from Alcoholics Anonymous: "Live your life one day at a time."

I think I'm getting there. Each day seems all the more precious. It's a gift to be savored. I awoke this morning enthusiastic.

◆━━━◆◆◆◆◆◆◆━━━◆

There's good news on the battlefront! The American Cancer Society is reporting dropping rates of new prostate cancer and declining mortality rates!

It is apparent now that we were finding ever more prostate cancers between 1989 and 1992 because PSA testing was spreading across the land. Those four years had the characteristics of an epidemic. Once we found all those men with unsuspected cancers and moved them into therapy, the number of new cases was bound to plummet. The Society estimates new cases for 2000 will fall to about 180,000 men.

The Society also estimates deaths will fall to 32,000 men in the year 2000. That reflects a falling rate of 2.5% annually since 1992. We must be doing something right!

Other good news: According to *Cancer Facts And Figures:*

⇨ Seventy-nine percent of all prostate cancers are discovered in the local and regional stages. The five-year relative survival rate for patients whose tumors are diagnosed at these stages is 100%.

⇨ Over the past twenty years, the (five-year) survival rate for all stages combined has increased from 67% to 92%.

⇨ Survival after a diagnosis of prostate cancer continues to decline beyond five years. According to

213

the most recent data, 67% of men diagnosed with prostate cancer survive 10 years, and 52% survive 15 years.

⇨ Prostate cancer accounts for 29% of men's cancer; it accounts for only 11% of their cancer related deaths. It's twice as common as the runner-up, lung cancer's 14%, but lung cancer is the major killer causing 31% of cancer related deaths. The figures are similar for women's breast cancer vs. lung cancer.

When I speak to a man with new prostate cancer, there's an unspoken question always lurking in the background: *Will I be able to have normal sex again?* My therapy rendered me impotent for about eighteen months. Sexual function has returned, but it's not like the good old days. Thank God for Viagra!

The implications of impotence are enormous from a man's perspective! American society places great value on a man's prowess in bed. The media is rife with sexual innuendo—if not downright exploitation. This culture defines a man by his career (therefore his income), his sexual charisma (including his athletic talent), the woman on his arm and the car he drives. Other considerations such as the philosophy he lives, his dedication to his family, his ethics, sensitivity, valor and patriotism are only secondary. A man's intelligence and education carries import, but that's primarily related to his earning potential. Unfortunately many of us have bought into this nonsense. Do you think it a coincidence that the words potentate, potential, and potency all spring from the same root? It's a source of incredible embarrassment to be impotent in America! I was there! I felt it! And I was fortunate in my impotence. It was temporary, and I felt secure in my relationship with Sherry. I knew we'd somehow cope.

One fact about radiation therapy continues to nag me: Unlike the immediate effects of surgery, the impotence of radiation therapy takes time to manifest. It arrives on cat feet, sometimes years later, causing a progressive loss of sexual capacity. Radiation damages those blood vessels supplying a man's penis. Without a good blood flow, a penis will never become engorged. My short-lived impotence was begot by hormonal therapy. I appreciate that I am vulnerable to radiation induced vascular injury. I could once again become impotent. I've accepted that. I chose my therapy, attempting to minimize impotence. Now I'm compelled to play the cards that fall my way.

Some of the most poignant letters I've seen on The Circle have been from *women* struggling with their lost sexuality because of their partners' impotence. These women have had to deal with their own fears of loss—of losing their spouse, best friend, confidant, and lover. They have anxieties over loneliness and financial ruin. They must cope with their partners' mood swings, self-absorp-

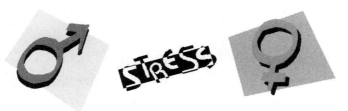

215

tion, new dietary needs, physical disabilities, and even deformities. They share their partners' periodic PSA anxiety. Now impotence falls into this roiling caldron of witches' brew! It can all be overwhelming. A woman often doesn't know what to expect or what options are available.

The topic of impotence is delicate. Anyone attempting a frank discussion runs the risk of offending someone. One can quickly be labeled a pervert, or at least preoccupied with sex. Strange, that sexual activity, so germane to our happiness, can be so delicate to discuss, particularly when the media and our culture assault us daily with exploited images of its reality! This subject is important! I intend to risk the accusations and have an honest conversation here.

Erectile dysfunction is the politically correct term these days. How I deplore that term; but Bob Dole uses it! There's only one good reason I can see for such obtuse verbiage: we can discuss it in front of the kids. (Or during Viagra commercials.) The kids will have no idea what we are talking about, and neither will 90% of the population.

Our pelvis has a rich nerve supply. I recall my days as a freshman medical student. My anatomy professor threw a surprise question into his exam: "Please diagram the nerve and blood supply of the male pelvis." I panicked! I remembered an anatomical drawing from Grey's Anatomy textbook. It seemed to show nerves and vessels everywhere! How could anyone remember such complexity? I had to portray something, or this exam would go down in flames.

With creative flamboyance I sketched the pelvic organs, and then illustrated nerves and blood vessels everywhere. What the hell, nothing ventured, nothing gained! The professor loved it! He commented to the class as he returned our papers: "Mr. Dorso fully realizes how complex is the neurovascular supply to the pelvis." I presume he was more amused than impressed with my work.

Anything injuring that rich array of nerves and blood vessels renders a man impotent. Radiation or surgical therapy can wreak havoc on those structures, but it's not by any means the only cause of impotence. Other illnesses, such as diabetes mellitus or hormonal diseases, can reduce a man's potency. Some medicines are notorious for causing impotence, especially those for controlling high blood pressure.

Impotence also comes with aging. That's expected, but not inevitable. Let's face it, nothing else works as well at 70 years as it did at 21!

Good statistics dealing with sexuality are hard to find. Statistics about a man's ability to perform in bed are suspect. Most of us are just not honest here. Probably twenty million U.S. men are impotent. It's a huge sub rosa epidemic.

My personal foray into a life of impotence began with my hormonal therapy. I had always enjoyed a healthy sexuality. It was hard for me to understand why some men couldn't get it up. I would merely contemplate embracing my lady, and there it was—no conscious effort required! I had looked forward to becoming a sexy senior citizen. Impotence was not in my life plan. John Lennon said it best: "Life is what happens while we're making plans." So true.

My impotence sneaked up on me like a thief in the night. About six weeks after I began hormonal therapy, my penis just gradually stopped working! I had a concomitant drop in libido, but I was sustained by my hope that this was all temporary. So I wasn't alarmed—not to worry.

After my seeding, my penis began to lose sensation. For a while the head of my penis was almost numb. I *knew* the nerves had taken a hit! Fortunately, that subsided over three months; although some loss of sensation persists to this day. I've been told that the nerves coursing along the surface of the prostate gland serve only to control the blood vessels of the penis. They control a man's erection through their ability to alter that blood flow. They carry no sensory nerves; therefore a man with a prostatectomy can expect normal sensation to his penis, even if his surgeon did not spare the nerves. I presume sensory nerves somewhere were also caught in the radiation crossfire.

Sherry and I went through a moratorium on our sexuality—that just seemed to happen without much discussion. As we gradually realized that impotence might be a permanent part of our lives, we began to clumsily discuss our options. Such discussions are not easy. We began to settle into a life of reduced sexuality—all the while hoping that some function would return as my body recovered from therapy. We continued to share our intimate moments, and supported each other with touching and hugs. In October, six months post seeding and four months after my last Lupron, I made a journal entry:

> It finally happened! Sherry and I managed to have intercourse for the first time in almost a year. I managed to muster up an erection that is best described as barely stuffable, but it worked! It was a triumph! My orgasm was dry. That was OK. It was still pleasurable. 'Pleasurable'! Hell, it was wonderful! As Sherry and I lie in each other's arms that night, the world was right again!

A few attempts at intercourse later that week were frustrating. I simply could not rise to the occasion. I began to realize that I would have to consider some sort of sexual aid if we were to have intercourse with any reliability.

By then I had heard of **Muse**, a new prescription medicine. This tiny tablet of Alprostadil (Prostaglandin E) is actually a miniature suppository. It's inserted into the urethra at the end of the penis. I approached Dr. Barnhill about it, and he gave me an instructional video. As he wrote a prescription for six tablets, he told me, "Since you seem to have some erectile function, you may not need a strong formulation. The suppository comes in strengths ranging from 250 milligrams to 1000 milligrams. We'll try the 250's and see how it goes."

I felt a sense of excitement as I stopped at the drug store for my new magic bullet. I was a bit embarrassed when presenting my prescription for penile urethral suppositories at the drug counter. Ever notice that those counters seem perpetually staffed by young women? My embarrassment quickly turned to frustration when I learned that six suppositories would cost me $120.00, and my HMO would not pay for the medicine! I presume they don't consider a healthy sexual life necessary for my well being.

It doesn't take a rocket scientist to realize that this love potion will cost me twenty dollars a pop. At that rate, sex once weekly would cost over a thousand dollars yearly. I later complained to a bachelor colleague, about the high cost of love these days. After reflecting a bit he exclaimed: "Hell, I've spent a lot more than that on sex! Just calculate the annual cost of dinners, drinks, shows, condoms, cologne and hotel rooms."

The Muse video was well done. Cartoon figures showed how to insert the tiny pill an inch into my penis. The cartoon man then rolled his cartoon penis between his cartoon hands for about ten seconds to dissolve the pill. An anonymous voice in the background was giving instructions. He told me that I could expect an erection in about ten minutes, and that some men experienced a "slight burning." If the burning was troublesome, I could relieve the burning by massaging my penis. Looked pretty simple!

I could see that this might not be so bad. I pictured myself that evening with my lady. I would excuse myself to the bathroom, and discreetly slip a tiny pill into my penis. Ten minutes later I would be a stud again—just like old times!

I was home alone that afternoon. I was supposed to be napping in preparation for a midnight shift. This was a perfect opportunity to see how I could strut my stuff.

A few minutes later I had one of those tiny pills in my penis. As I rolled my penis in my hands, I could feel a burning sensation beginning in my urethra. No problem! The video had warned me that "Some men experienced a slight burning." Following instructions, I rolled some more. The burning got worse. I ignored it. Keep rolling! Then, just like clockwork at ten minutes, my penis stiffened into a natural looking erection. Yea Gods! It looked great! There was only one problem: It burned like hell!

Now I was in proud possession of an erect burning poker! No pun intended. More rolling didn't help! Still more discomfort—now radiating to my scrotum! I tried to ignore it and go to sleep. Easier to ignore Godzilla. There would be no sleep with this going on! I had to get rid of this stiff, burning penis!

The burning finally moved me to action. I ran outside and jumped into the hot tub. That seemed to help—only a little bit. Finally in desperation I urinated into the hot water. Ahhhhh, blessed relief came over the next few minutes. Flushing the medicine out of my urethra was the solution! I sat there in the tub as the water swirled about me brooding, "Here sits Doctor Dorso: An old man, home alone, penis on fire, peeing in his hot tub! What a sex life!"

The next day after I drained and refilled the tub, I went to see Dr. Barnhill. He grinned briefly and confided, "I was wondering how you would do. I've heard complaints about penile burning from some of my patients. I've noticed that patient requests for refills of Muse seemed to taper off with time."

It was a couple of weeks before I mustered the courage to try the Muse again—this time with Sherry. The second time produced much less burning, but my erection was useless. Pondering what had happened, I finally read the instructions with care.

Muse is unstable. The shelf life is only two weeks at room temperature. The druggist mentioned that I should store it in the refrigerator. I didn't plan to store it; I planned to *use it*! Because I did not relish explaining what this stuff was to anyone poking about the refrigerator, I kept it in my bedside drawer, and it lost its punch. I didn't realize it could happen so fast.

I finally came to a disappointing appraisal. Muse was not for me. For some reason it produces intolerable burning in my urethra. It's expensive. It's unstable. Not willing to risk another hassle, I chucked the package into the trash.

A couple of confidants advised me to try **"the pump."** Actually it's a vacuum device that will produce an erection with virtually any penis. I called Osbon Medical Systems (1-800-438-8592). When I identified myself as an author they shipped a complimentary, battery powered Esteem model. It seemed a bit pricey at $500.00, but was well thought-out and constructed. Some models are much cheaper. Rumor has it that the original developer was once under investigation by the Postal Service for shipping obscene materials. Enlightenment does come slowly.

My pump came with a graphic instructional video. A man in the film put his penis into a transparent cylinder held firmly to his body. As the pump sucked out the cylinder's air, his penis filled with blood and grew to full length. He put a tight rubber band about the base of his penis and removed the cylinder. Voila! A functional erection.

We used the pump a few times, and it worked. Fortunately, about that time, my own function was recovering and the pump was gradually relegated to the bottom drawer of my bedside table. I found it distracting to interpose this artificial device into the middle of our lovemaking, but we adapted. I suspect I would be content to continue with my pump if I had to.

I never got around to trying penile injection therapy. This has been around for about twenty years. I've heard that the physician developing the technique couldn't get any attention from the medical establishment, until he did a live demonstration on himself—on stage! Various drugs injected into the penis will produce a high quality erection in about 70% of the men trying it. Caverject (alprostadil) is a popular name. It even comes with an automatic injector! I think I would have been able to get past my needle phobia, if necessary. The cost per injection is somewhere between $5.00 and $20.00, depending on the prescription. Once again the cost of love could approach $1,000.00 yearly!

———————

I was not surprised when my sexual capacities began to fade six weeks after starting Lupron and Casodex. I was **astounded** when I realized that I really didn't seem to miss the sex. Intellectually, I knew that I would enjoy sexual intercourse, but I didn't have that insistent, instinctive, grinding feeling in my gut that sporadically demanded attention.

I had always considered my sexuality to be an integral part of who I was. Now I realize that part of who "**I**" was depended upon a few drops of testosterone produced daily in my groin. Those precious drops of love potion not only generated my sexual appetite: They grew my muscles, controlled my weight, begot body hair, added an aggressive, competitive edge to my behavior, created stamina, provoked erections.

I have to ask, what other aspects of myself are really the result of biological imperatives? **Who is my core person?** Great thinkers throughout history have examined that question.

Marcus Aurelius pondered it. He found time during his campaign against the barbarians in 167 AD to write his *Meditations*. He said it so eloquently:

> Try to see, before it is too late, that you have within you something higher and more godlike than mere instincts which move your emotions

and twitch you like a puppet. Which of these is it then, that is clouding my understanding at this moment? Fear, jealousy, lust, or some other?

A modern poet, Hugh Prather, said it with remarkable precision, "Anyone who inhabits himself cannot believe in objective thinking."

I enjoy Goethe's *Faust*, the classic story in which Faust sells his soul to the devil, Mephisto. Mephisto, masquerading as a college professor, gives advice to an eager student:

> How do you study something living?
> Drive out the spirit, deny it being,
> So there's just parts with which to deal,
> Gone is that anomalous thing, the soul.
> With lifeless pieces the only things real,
> The wonder's where's the life of the whole.

Desmond Morris wrote *The Naked Ape* in 1967. He's a zoologist, who seems to have taken Mephisto's advice and done away with the soul entirely. He sees mankind as just a flourishing ape:

> There are one hundred and ninety-three living species of monkeys and apes. One hundred and ninety-two of them are covered with hair. The exception is a naked ape self named Homo Sapiens. This unusual and highly successful species spends a great deal of time examining his higher motives and an equal amount of time studiously ignoring his fundamental ones. He is proud that he has the biggest brain of all the primates, but attempts

conceal the fact that he also has the biggest
ɔnis, preferring to accord this honor falsely to
ᴜᴇ mighty gorilla…

In acquiring lofty new motives, he has lost
none of the earthy old ones. This is frequently
a cause of some embarrassment to him, but his
old impulses have been with him for millions
of years, his new ones only a few thousand at
the most—and there is no hope of quickly
shrugging off the accumulated genetic legacy
of his whole evolutionary past. He would be a
far less worried and more fulfilled animal if
only he would face up to this fact.

As for me, the truth lies somewhere in the middle
ground. Marcus has it almost right for me. Our inner
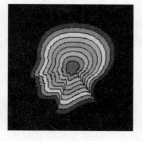 being—call it soul, spirit, or ego—
resides in a physical body, which
compels us to meet its own needs.
Marcus would have us rise above our
physical impulses, and gain control
over those passions, which cloud our
judgement. Too many people today would have us completely ignore our passions. What a great formula for
unhappiness! I agree with Desmond's contention that we
need to face up to our genetic legacy. The healthy individual has accepted that part of his nature, and integrated
it into his personality. Good old Popeye had it right with
his exclamation, "I yam what's I Yam!"

As I watched the feminization of my body, complete

with developing breasts, I went into a mild depression. I'm convinced that it was mild only because I knew most of this would reverse itself after therapy. If I were forced to endure such hormonal therapy for the rest of my life, I have no doubt that I would have to deal with a significant depression. (And, who knows, I may still have to go there if this cancer refuses to behave.)

I found succor in the arms of my wife. She was always there for me. I admit that I actually became a bit clinging. I suspect that some men have trouble expressing physical affection, except during sexual play. Take away their sexuality, and they're at a loss for what a hug is supposed to mean. I was fortunate. I was part of a loving family where there was touching, hugging, demonstrative affection. It was easy for me to enjoy the therapeutic benefits of loving touch with my entire family.

I really miss my prostate gland! Let's face it, I destroyed mine. (Some people choose to cut it out.) In the beginning of this book, I described the prostate's function as producing 80% of a man's semen. That's a proper doctoral thing to say. What I didn't realize is that it produces about 80% of the pleasure of an ejaculation. That feel-good pulsing in my groin during orgasm is gone! Instead there is a brief, vague discomfort coming from that poor, atrophic, irritated, irradiated prostate gland as it dutifully tries to respond in a hurts-so-good motif.

And of course the orgasms are dry. Gone are the orgasmic waves of contractions through my genitalia producing this vital life's fluid. That's one more sensation I'll never again experience.

I've also had to deal with an irritable bladder. Mine wasn't happy being caught in the radiation bathing my pelvis. It now seems to register **full** at three ounces, and with unseemly insistence. That makes it difficult to sit through a movie or more than a hundred miles in a car. A shopping trip has to be planned with a pit stop in mind. I'm certainly becoming aware of where all the bathrooms are in town.

I'm taking a new drug, **Flomax**. (Isn't that a great name? You just know what Flomax is for!) My prostate gland has periods of spasm—usually during the night—and with its hold on my urethra, can make urination difficult. Flomax has largely replaced Cardura and Hytrin for that purpose. Its advantage is that it has minimal effect on a man's blood pressure. (Both Hytrin and Cardura are blood pressure pills.) Flomax's disadvantage is that it costs more. Some health plans don't want to pay for it unless a patient is having unwanted symptoms of low blood pressure—such as becoming light-headed when getting out of a chair—when using either Hytrin or Cardura.

My rectum shows some radiation effects as well. My gut just seems more irritable. My once daily B.M. has become two or three. I've learned to avoid hot spicy foods. Too much fruit can wreak havoc. My doctors repeatedly ask if I'm having any rectal bleeding. Fortunately, I've been able to say no.

Erections are usually serviceable. Viagra makes a big difference. We use it periodically, for special occasions. Because Viagra needs time to work, I have to anticipate events an hour ahead of time. It's expensive at $8.00 a pill. God forbid that my eight dollar ship of hope should wreck on the shoals of an unexpected headache. And Viagra gives me a stuffy nose. Honest! The same mechanism that causes penile swelling can cause nasal membranes to swell. So now I have to balance my desire for sexual stamina against my desire for sleep without snoring. I used the larger dose of 100 milligrams (instead of 50 milligrams) for a while, and the nasal congestion was even worse.

Because Viagra affects the production of visual pigments in one's eyes, the 100 milligram dose has a peculiar effect of creating a blue tint everywhere I look. There also seems to be an immutable Viagra law of the universe: The youngest woman in the pharmacy is the one who will hand you your prescription.

Forty-nine men died last year for every one million prescriptions of Viagra. That's compared to 1.5 deaths per million prescriptions of Muse. Something may be going on. Most men don't seem to care. Frankly, I don't. Not bad odds. Forty-nine to a million. I'll take those odds if I can enjoy a sexual life! We already know that taking nitroglycerine with Viagra can be fatal. Me? I avoid nitroglycerine. Dr. Jerry Avorn, at Boston's Brigham and Women's Hospital says:

"If you find old guys on Viagra dying from heart attacks, it's hard to know if it's the Viagra or the sexual activity. But that doesn't mean we shouldn't try to find out."

In March, 2000, researchers from Cedars-Sinai Medical Center gave an unsettling report to the American College of Cardiologists in Anaheim, CA. They analyzed 1,473 FDA reports of adverse effects of Viagra. Five hundred and twenty-two of those people died, probably from cardiovascular causes. These were not all "old guys!" Most were less than 65 years of age, without knowledge of heart disease, and were taking a prescribed dose of Viagra. Ninety men suffered heart problems because they mixed Viagra and nitroglycerine.

I presume most of these men had engaged in sexual intercourse. That fact seems to be left out of the picture sometimes! In case you haven't noticed, sex makes a man's heart rate and blood pressure rise. It involves significant cardiovascular activity.

In some countries where prostitution is legal, (and cheap), and drugs unregulated, men are dying in even bigger numbers from Viagra overdose; as they attempt two or three trysts a day. I suspect there are American men so desperate for sexual performance that they are also overdosing.

As of press time, the issue remains unsettled. My advice to my readers is to keep an ear tuned to the news about Viagra. Discuss it with your doctor. Don't risk an extra pill to improve performance. Don't ever take nitroglycerine if you use Viagra.

My private concern is that the FDA will decide the drug is dangerous and pull it off the market! At which point pushers will become rich smuggling Viagra at exorbitant prices! I've heard stories of Viagra selling for as much as $80.00 a tablet in some countries where it's still illegal.

——————◄•••••••►——————

So, despite the grousing, I haven't a great deal to complain about. Sex isn't the same as it was at age twenty-one. But then few other bodily functions are either. We've adapted, and enjoy a fulfilling, mature sexual life. I submit that it becomes a different, deeper expression of one's sexuality when we must communicate through our older bodies, our more vulnerable bodies, our less power-oriented, less invincible bodies. We're forced to love with heightened tenderness, more words, more silence, even more silliness; more counting of precious moments that are driven by a whole, human passion for one another.

So why does it feel as if I'm complaining? I think the answer appears when I look at my tattoos. I have three tattooed blue spots: one for each thigh and one over my pubic bone—three silent reminders of what I've been through. That's really the rub for all cancer survivors. We're all trying to lead a normal life; trying not to look back—Death may be gaining on us. Now even the expression of love brings a reminder that things are not normal, that I have cancer, that I'm closer to death than a man my age should have to be.

Expressing one's sexuality is difficult when the Grim Reaper sends flowers for the bedroom.

———————

An important study came out of the Fred Hutchinson Research Center in Seattle in January, 2000. They discovered that impotency among men electing radical prostatectomies was greater than had been previously reported! Surprised?

These people did yeoman service producing this mega-study. They followed 1,291 men who were randomly selected from bread and butter hospitals scattered across six states. They intentionally avoided the high volume medical centers. They wanted a sampling of the care received by most Americans. They went through all those medical records to ensure that the biopsy and staging was correct. They polled the patients every six months. Mean age at diagnosis was 63 years. The authors note, "Most patients were white, married, high school or college educated, and retired."

At eighteen months post surgery, 60% of the men studied "reported that erections were not firm enough for sexual intercourse, and 44% were unable to have any erections." The nerve-sparing surgery helped a bit: 56% of those men with both nerves saved reported impotence versus 66% of those with non-nerve sparing surgery.

And how did these men cope with their impotence?

"During the 24 month follow-up, these treatments were used: vacuum suction device, 26.8%; penile injections, 21.4%; medication, 9.0%; counseling by a sex therapist or psychologist, 7.6%; and penile implant or prosthesis, 3.7%."

They also reported that 8% were incontinent of urine, and 16% needed surgery for strictures.

The most amazing thing to me is on the last page of the seven-page report:

"Despite the level of urinary incontinence and sexual dysfunction...most men (75.5%) were satisfied or pleased with their treatment, and most (71.5%) would choose radical prostatectomy again."

Dr. P. Walsh, et. al, from the James Buchanan Urological Institute of Johns Hopkins Medical Institutions have presented a paper in *Urology* (Jan 2000) describing their results. Surgeons there followed sixty-four men for the eighteen months after nerve sparing radical prostatectomy (for localized prostate cancer). These men were all potent prior to surgery. They defined "**potency**" as the ability to have unassisted intercourse *with or without Viagra*. By eighteen months, 86% were potent, and 84% considered *"sexual bother"* as none or small. (Sexual bother! Now there's a euphemism a Wall Street advertiser could use with pride!)

They defined "urinary continence" as the ability to live without wearing pads, and report that 93% of their patients were dry. (Which corresponds with results in the previous report.)

How can two studies be reporting impotency rates that are so divergent? For one thing, Johns Hopkins is one of the preeminent surgical Centers in the world—especially for prostate cancer—and Dr. Walsh is one of the most renowned surgeons. This is as good as it gets! If you consider radical prostatectomy for your care, go to a center of excellence such as this.

⎯⎯•◦●◉●◦•⎯⎯

I do periodic PSA's to follow my progress. Every survivor of prostate cancer does. I commented earlier, that living with cancer is like trying to live with (and ignore) a rhinoceros in the room. When it's time to do another PSA, that rhino becomes almost palpable. I can feel the background tension beginning to rise as I await **The Number**, like some pronouncement from On High. I've come to realize that there are as many as two million men in this country who live from PSA to PSA. Two million families building their hopes around an impersonal lab slip, a ticket to life, that tallies the days their loved one may coexist on this orb. "May you have many low PSAs" has become a common salutation among survivors of prostate cancer.

My PSA plummeted to less than 0.1 within months of my first Lupron injection, and stayed there. Dr. Blasko was so enthusiastic with my first annual exam that he advised me to relax, and just do the PSA every six months. Six months later my PSA had risen to 0.6! Trying not to panic, I called Dr. Blasko. His nurse, Alea, calmed my fears.

"About a third of our patients have a mild rise in PSA levels at eighteen months. So far, there seems to be no correlation between 'benign PSA rises' and treatment failure. Relax, and repeat the PSA in two months."

She sent excerpts from Dr. Blasko's book, *Prostate Brachytherapy Made Complicated*, (Don't you just love that title!) in which he writes:

> Benign PSA rises occur commonly between 12 and 24 months following implantation (of seeds)... The prognosis for such patients appears good. While there is currently no precise explanation for benign PSA rises after brachytherapy, their frequent occurrence is something to be aware of. Because of many patients' tendency to panic with any PSA rise, they should be warned in advance of the possibility of a benign PSA rise. Patients need to be reassured that it is not a significant event. (Who, ME?)

Dr. John Blasko knew what he was talking about. Two months later, my PSA was once again safely below 0.1! It's still there—three years post therapy.

In the spring of 2000, Dr. John Blasko released some nine-year results. This was significant for three reasons:

⇨ There are few studies that run this long.

⇨ Most brachytherapy studies are using radioactive iodine (I-125) seeds. This one reports results with radioactive Palladium (Pd-103) and discusses the differences.

⇨ All were treated with Pd-103 as the **only** treatment—no surgery, hormone suppression, or other radiation.

He studied 230 men with "clinically organ confined disease" (roughly stages A & B) over nine years. (Since men have been continually entering the study, the median follow-up is now 41.5 months.)

He comments that because Pd-103 is a hotter isotope, it may confer an advantage to men with more malignant disease. "For this reason, patients with (more malignant disease) were more likely to be selected for treatment with Pd-103." Bottom line: he didn't select just the easy cases.

Dr. Blasko avoids the word "cure," and instead refers to "biochemical control." He defines treatment failure as two successive rises in PSA, or otherwise obvious clinical recurrence—such as a growing, hard prostate gland on rectal examination, or x-ray evidence of spread to the bones or other organs.

To date, 199 men are apparently free of disease, and no patient in this series has died of prostate cancer!

In this study, he found two risk factors that reduce a man's chance of cure:

+ PSA over 10

+ Gleason Score 7 or above

When these risk factors were taken into consideration, five years after seeding:

+ 94% of the men show biochemical control if they have neither risk factor

+ 82% with one risk factor

+ 65% with both risk factors

Patterns became apparent as he watched those men enrolled early in the program. Dr Blasko can now mathematically predict how all his patients will do over nine years. *He predicts 83.5% of his 230 patients will be living with no evidence of disease, nine years after therapy.* That's 192 men virtually cured!

Patients with more advanced or more aggressive disease do not have as great a chance for cure regardless of whether the treatment is surgery or seed implants.

As I ponder these figures I am both encouraged and chagrined—encouraged because I have good odds for personal survival, chagrined because I allowed my PSA to rise from 10 to about 15. That prolonged period of denial allowed my own five-year odds to slip. Of course these figures do not apply to me, because I had external beam radiation as well as seed implants, and I endured eight months of hormone suppression therapy. Nevertheless, this is an encouraging study!

The take-home lessons we can learn here:

- Take heart! Your chances for long-term survival are excellent.

- Do whatever you must to keep your PSA from rising early in the game.

- Consider hormonal suppression therapy if you intend to spend time examining your options.

Cancer, for me, was a wake up call. I had been living my life as if I had forever. Life had become a bit too comfortable. I would have been content to drift along,

237

working my shifts, paying my mortgage, raising four wonderful children, taking my share of vacations, gardening in my spare time. I seemed productively engaged, but I was postponing much of the inner work of life. I was distracted from some of life's deeper meaning by life itself. I had always intended to read the Bible—some day. I often dreamed of visiting Alaska—some day. I planned to get more involved in spiritual study—some day.

I had envisioned a contemplative life in my "Golden Years." Then I would be relieved of the burden of going to work on a daily basis, while living in an empty nest. Life would have a slower pace. I just *expected* a healthy, old age of many years.

It's easy to be distracted in modern America. The media provides us endless opportunities. There's the latest movie to see, the news at ten, the paper in the morning with a couple cups of coffee, e-mail to check, catalogues in the mail, the web to surf. Then there's hospital meetings, hobbies, medical conventions, reports to write, bills to pay, investments to monitor, grass to mow, cars to wash, dogs to walk. We are awash in information and "factoids," much of it repetitive, banal, useless—distractions all!

Who cares who shot whom in the neighboring town! Why does anyone watch an hour's program about how the movie stars live? If I were a fallen angel opposing humankind's inner development, this is how I would do it: turn America into a nation of automatons busily distracted from their true purpose in life.

And purposeful activity is not bad! Hobbies are not bad! My hobby is astronomy. It provides meditative time and companionship. When I'm contemplating the inconceivable size and numbers of the universe, I'm awestruck. What wondrous power was required to create this grandeur! At these moments, I find myself as close to my Creator as I have ever been.

Cancer was a shot across my bow. Time to examine my ship's course! In fact, time is what we're talking about here. Cancer suddenly made me aware that time is a limited resource. Of course, it's always been a limited quantity for all of us, but that reality was now suddenly in my face. Life is ephemeral!

Shakespeare said it so well, *"We are such stuff as dreams are made of."*

One day I had to ask myself: "Self, you are now in your late fifties, when are you really going to read that Bible, when are you going to join that study group, and do you truly intend to see Alaska? And, by the way, when is the last time you went out of your way to make a difference in someone's life? When did you last read a challenging, thought-provoking book, visit a shut-in, volunteer for a community effort?"

No time? Of course not! There's a new animated Disney movie to see!

This book came out of such self-examination. This is one attempt to make a difference, to give something back to society. It hasn't been easy to be so frank about the intimate details of my life. I'm feeling vulnerable here!

Writing a book certainly exposes me to possible criticism, but cancer has given me a special perspective on vulnerability. Once a man has been spread-eagled in stirrups with twenty-two needles in his crotch, vulnerability has new meaning. I thought about writing this book anonymously, but feared it would lose some of its credibility. I chose to be vulnerable.

I planted a seed of hope when I wrote this book. It's been a long time a-borning! It's my hope that it will make a difference in the lives of many men and their families. Of course we all plant seeds of hope! Don't we expect to harvest something from the rich experiences of parenthood, work, marriage, success, and failure? Don't we have countless opportunities to REAP, to HARVEST, to GLEAN meaning from life's experiences?

Illness is just such a rich experience! I doubt that any of us would have chosen cancer! Our only choice now is how to respond. It's important to plant your own seeds of hope here. I challenge you to look at your own life in the wake of your own experience of this disease. This will take courage, but I have confidence in the resiliency of the human spirit. Expect to harvest something meaningful from this experience, to walk away enriched. The alternative is to limp away from this kind of illness battered and beaten.

I've discovered many personal *seeds of hope* as I've lived through my story. I've learned that opening myself to new expressions of love and intimacy is another way to be vulnerable. I've discovered that honestly communi-

240

cating what lives in my heart can produce real transformation—not only self-transformation, but transformation in my relationships. I've learned that I must be willing to let go of previous definitions of intimacy, to become vulnerable, and to be transformed in the process, to grow into someone new—not less, *new*. I've learned to put my trust in other human beings—be they cab drivers or physicians.

I've come to understand a person's embarrassment over his illness, and how important it is to offer some hope—regardless of how hopeless the situation seems to me as a physician. I've felt the separation inherent in any serious ailment. I've come to realize how easy it is to blame a patient for his or her infirmity. I've experienced my own denial and fears of medical procedures. I feel closer to my creator. I've accepted that my destiny is really in His hands. That's been a true catharsis in many respects. I've realized that we are indeed *all special*, but being special does not absolve us from suffering. What makes us special is how we bear up under the yoke of our suffering. I've been inspired by the story of Viktor Frankl, a psychiatrist who survived the death camps of Nazi Germany:

> The way in which man accepts his fate and all the suffering it entails, the way in which he takes up his cross, gives him an ample opportunity—even under the most difficult circumstances—to add a deeper meaning to his life. He may remain brave, dignified, and unselfish. Or in the bitter fight for self-preservation he may forget his human dignity and become no more than an animal. Here lies the chance for

a man either to make use of or to forgo the opportunities of attaining the moral values that a difficult situation may afford him. And this decides whether he is worthy of his sufferings or not.

I've accepted my mortality and acknowledged my frailty—both physical and emotional. I've discovered strengths I wasn't sure I had. I'm certainly more empathetic, not only as physician, but as a friend, father, spouse. I've learned the value of time, and the importance of culling out the busy from the real. I've chosen to spend more time with my family.

I still find it hard to take the time for play. I need to find more time for laughter.

I've learned that I can survive!

It is my sincere hope that you, my dear reader, will find your own path to survival, and that this book has offered you encouragement and strength. Although these pages chronicle my own research, therapeutic choices, and my course through the labyrinth of prostate cancer, I cannot deny the success of other men who have taken different paths. My purpose here has been to humbly share what the journey has been for me.

Trust your instincts, then do everything you can to maximize your choice.

You too can survive!

May you find your own seeds of hope.

May you have many low PSAs.

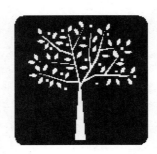

We must eradicate from the soul all fear and terror
of what comes to meet us from the future.
We must look forward with absolute equanimity
to whatever comes,
and we must think that whatever comes is given to us
by a world direction full of wisdom.
It is part of what we must learn in this age,
namely, to act out of pure trust
in the ever present help of the spiritual world.
Truly, nothing else will do,
if our courage is not to fail us.
Let us discipline our will;
and let us seek the awakening from within ourselves
every morning and every evening.

—Rudolph Steiner

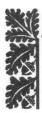

RESOURCES:
FOR MEN WITH PROSTATE CANCER &
THE MEN AND WOMEN WHO LOVE THEM?

The American Cancer Society, 1-800-227-2345
This is of course the Big Daddy of volunteer organizations
with two million volunteers, a professional staff of 4,418
working in over 3400 local unit and division offices, and 463
people in the national home office! The Society has invested
over $2 billion in cancer research and provided grant support
to 30 Nobel Prize winners. Because of that, I've listed them
first. To catalogue all they offer would require another book.
Suffice it to say that volunteers are available to offer support
and information at all hours. You can order their book,
Prostate Cancer, by phone. Visit their web site at
http://www.cancer.org

The Cancer Information Service, 1-800-422-6237
(That's 1-800-4 cancer.)
This rich resource is a service of The National Cancer
Institute, the nation's primary agency for cancer research.
Their mission is to "provide the latest and most accurate
cancer information to patients and their families, the public,
and health professionals."Their staff of "information specialists" fields 500,000 calls annually. Open 24x7, they answer
calls in Spanish and English, and can accommodate the
hearing impaired or deaf caller with TTY equipment at 1-
800-332-8615. Visit the information web site at
http://www.nci.nih.gov and click on the Information Service
Link.

Patient Advocates For Advanced Cancer Treatment,
1-616-453-1477
The philosophy of the organization seems to discourage both
radical prostatectomy and radiation therapy. They see prostate

cancer as a systemic disease early in its course, and encourage intermittent hormonal suppression therapy, and herbal therapy around PC SPES. They publish a quarterly Cancer Communication Newsletter available by phone, or on-line, http://www.osz.com/paact.

The Cancer Hotline,
1-800-433-0464
Twenty-two years ago Mr. Bloch was diagnosed with "ter-minal" lung cancer, and given a short time to live. This is the same Mr. Bloch of H&R Block, (He Anglicized the spelling for business purposes.) who is obviously a man of action. He's still a survivor! He and his wife Annette "dedicated their lives to helping the next person who gets cancer" by gener-ously funding the R.A. Bloch Cancer Foundation, and writing three books: *Fighting Cancer, Guide for Cancer Supporters*, and *Cancer...There's Hope*. The books and a phone call to order them are free. They offer other forms of support as well. Their website is http://www.blochcancer.org

Urologic Foundation Information Hotline,
1-800-242-2383
A call will require you to wend your way through a list of menus, often ending with a voice mail option; but they do offer educational material on impotence, and prostate cancer.

Prostate Cancer Awareness Pins
Rick Ward is a survivor of prostate cancer. One of his mis-sions is to provide lapel pins for those wishing to increase awareness of prostate cancer. The pin resembles a blue ribbon. It's an attractive blue with gold colored outline—about an inch long. Rick has made them available at his cost. You can order them on the internet, pcapin@prodigy.net Order them by the dozen for $5.05 including postage and packaging. Give them to all your friends and doctors! I sus-pect he's losing money on this project. I have no doubt that he would appreciate any donation to support his effort.

Help Yourself, 1-318-396-4440
Tracy Moore is another survivor of prostate cancer who saw a need for an informative video. He has a created a fifty-

minute video outlining even more resources. He has created a non-profit organization, Xylomed Research, dedicated to research with plant medicinals. His newsletter is now in its 9th year of publication. Use the above number to order the video for $25.00. E-mail him at trmoore@bayou.com

Proton Beam Therapy, 1-909-824-4378
If you're considering proton beam therapy, call Loma Linda University in Southern California. They have an informative web page, info@proton.llumc.edu

CAPCURE, 1-800-757-2873 (That's 1-800-757-CURE)
Michael Milken is a nationally recognized name in invest-ment circles, and was diagnosed with incurable prostate cancer. He founded this organization with a generous grant, dedicated to finding a cure for prostate cancer. Access their web page at, http://www.capcure.org for information—espe-cially for outstanding dietary advice.

Theragenics, 1-770-271-0233
These are the people who make the radioactive "Theraseeds" for brachytherapy. The company maintains an informative web page at http://www.theragenics.com offering information and literature about the procedure.

Seattle Prostate Institute, 1-206-215-2480
This is where you can find John C. Blasko, M.D. if you're interested in brachytherapy at a center of excellence. He's my guru!

FULL CIRCLE: RECOMMENDED READING

For this section, I turned to my own support group, *The Circle*. Informally called "Circlers," this group of men and women spans the globe and meets in cyberspace. An assembly of prostate cancer survivors and their significant others, Circlers have provided a rich source of support and knowledge for me. I naturally turned to their collective wisdom as I searched for recommended reading. The suggested reading list below is their list, compiled by me over the internet. I have put their comments in italics to set them apart from mine. The books are listed in no particular order of priority.

The ABC's Of Prostate Cancer; The Book That could Save Your Life
By Joseph E. Osterling, Mark A. Moyad, and Joseph E. Osterling; Paperback, 356 pages, 1997, ISBN 1568330979
"This was the first one to really help me early on. I found the chapter that stated this was a woman's disease too. I needed to hear that so much."
This book features messages of hope from over 50 well-known survivors of prostate cancer, including Bob Dole, Jerry Lewis, and Sidney Poitier.

Prostate and Cancer: A Family Guide To Diagnosis, Treatment, and Survival, Revised Edition
By Sheldon Marks, M.D., Paperback, 352 pages, 1999, ISBN 1555612067
This book is written in Question & Answer format in a larger type for aging eyes. It's now in its third revision and fifth printing—a staple in support groups.

The Prostate; A Guide For Men And The Women Who Love Them
By Patrick C. Walsh M.D. and Janet Farrar Worthington. Paperback, 480 pages, 1997, ISBN 0446604321
Dr. Walsh is a pre-eminent surgeon who developed the nerve-sparing radical prostatectomy. He presents well-balanced advice about effective forms of therapy.
"If you have not seen this, it is really worth the look."
"We used it only a little. Not much on aftercare."

The American Cancer Society: Prostate Cancer, Revised Edition
By David G. Bostwick, M.D., Gregory T. Maclennan, M.D., and Thayne R. Larson, M.D.
This book contains basic, essential information, clearly presented. It's billed as "A thorough and compassionate resource for patients and their families."

A Cancer Battle Plan; Six Strategies For Beating Cancer, from A Recovered Hopeless Case

By Anne E. Frahm, and David J. Frahm, contributor
Paperback 172 pages, Putnam Publishers, 1998,
ISBN 087477893x
"I started with A Battle Plan For Cancer. It's about Anne's battle with breast cancer. It was very interesting, and gave me hope that something could be done with prostate cancer."
Publisher's Comment: "Includes resource lists and a complete nutrition battle plan."

The Patient's Guide To Prostate Cancer; An Expert's Successful Treatment Strategies and Options

By Marc B. Garnick, 1996 paperback
Ron Koster is a Circler who weekly posts his list of recommended reading for The Circle. He orders them in priority. This is first on his list.
"The first book is a fast read and introduces the newcomer to most of what s/he wants to know. It's not very informative about brachytherapy or Proton Beam Therapy."

Prostate Cancer; A Non-surgical Perspective

By Kent Waller, M.D. Paperback 172 pages,
ISBN 0964899108, Large Print
Ron Koster's second recommendation:
"The second book is helpful on brachytherapy, and mentions Proton Beam. I simply haven't found a good book that does a good job on Proton Beam."

Love, Sex, and PSA: Living And Loving With Prostate Cancer

By Robert Hitchcox and Betty Wilson, Illustrator
Paperback, 109 pages, 1997, ISBN 0965973408
"The book that I found, before my surgery, that was very helpful for both myself and my wife in preparation for the surgery and its after-effects. Both of us enjoyed the book immensely. The humor came out at just the right time. The book also gave us a number of hints/ideas in preparing for surgery that neither of us had thought of."

The Herbal Remedy For Prostate Cancer
By James Lewis Jr., PhD, 1999, 216 pages, ISBN 1883257026
"About PC SPES, based on clinical trials. A good book!" PC SPES is an herbal preparation used for treatment of prostate cancer. This book tells how to do it, and lists possible side effects and remedies. (There is a support group on the internet for those men using this treatment option, which is listed in my book's Resource List.)

Revolutionary Approach To Prostate Cancer
By Dr Aubrey Pilgrim, 1997, 328 pages, ISBN 1563150867
Aubrey Pilgrim holds a Doctorate of Chiropractic Medicine, and is himself a survivor of prostate cancer. He's soon to release an expanded, revised edition. His book is now available on-line, and there's no charge for downloading the text. Just go to: www.prostatepointers.org/prostate/lay/apilgrim. The proceeds from his book support Patient Advocates for Advanced Cancer Treatments (PAACT)
"The author is a member of the club, and offers the pros and cons of all the treatments available. He also goes into detail about the common side effects of treatment and how to deal with them."

How We Die; Reflections On Life's Final Chapter
By Sherwin B. Nuland, 1996, ISBN 0679742441, available on audiocassette.
"This book is a frank and unsentimental explanation of what happens to body and mind as we expire. From accident and suicide to the more lingering illnesses, we can see what is happening. A patient and his family can be better prepared for the inevitability of death with some of this information. The author is an MD who has written other books on various medical subjects."

Final Gifts; Understanding the Special Awareness Needs and Communications of the Dying
By Maggie Callahan and Patricia Kelly, Paperback, 1997, 239 pages, available large print, ISBN 0553378767
The co-authors are hospice nurses who share their insights on death. They describe an altered state of consciousness entered by a dying person, in which s/he drifts between both worlds.

They've coined the term, Nearing death awareness, to describe that state. They give instruction to caregivers in how to recognize this state, and speak with the dying person as s/he tries to communicate his or her needs. This is an inspiring book! I recommend this and Nuland's book (above) to anyone caring for a terminally ill loved one.
"Excellent for end stages of prostate cancer and other illnesses—beneficial to patients, families, and providers."

Prostate Cancer; Making Survival Decisions
By Sylvan Meyer and Seymour C. Nash, M.D., 264 pages, 1994, ISBN 0226568571
Mr. Meyer is a journalist. Dr. Nash is his urologist.
"When Bob was diagnosed in the summer of 1995, one of our daughters sent us this book. We found it to be very informative. The book was published in 1994, so it may not be up to date on the most recent break-through events."

From This Moment On: A Guide For Those Most Recently Diagnosed With Cancer
By Arlene Cotter, 384 pages, 1999, Random House, ISBN 0375503099
Arlene Cotter overcame non-Hodgkin's lymphoma.
"One of the best books I've seen for the newly diagnosed and their loved ones. This book has obviously been written by someone who has been there and done that, and has grown and learned from the experience. I only wish that she had written it a few years earlier so that I could have seen it at the start of my journey."

Beating Cancer With Nutrition: Clinically Proven And Easy-To-Follow Strategies To Dramatically Improve Quality And Quantity Of Life And Chances For A Complete Remission
By Patrick Quillin, Ph.D., and Noreen Quillin, 250 pages, 1998, ISBN 0963837249
"Great information on supplements and recipes."

The What To Eat If You Have Cancer Cookbook; Over 100 Easy-To-Prepare Recipes For Patients And Their Families And Caregivers

By Maureen Keane, M.S. and Daniella Chace, M.S.,
Paperback, 140 pages, 1997, ISBN 0809231298
A companion to the authors' book, *What To Eat If You Have Cancer.*
"Great tasting recipes, mostly for people who are doing a traditional treatment such as surgery, radiation, or chemotherapy."

The Lovin' Ain't Over; The Couples Guide To Better Sex After Prostate Disease
By Ralph and Barbara Alterowitz, Paperback, 160 pages, 1999, ISBN 1883257034. Ralph Alterowitz is founding vice chair and former Director of The National Prostate Cancer Coalition.
"This is a newer one, and I wish I had it from the beginning, as it is clear, concise, funny, and written by a couple—practical advice about lovemaking."

Man To Man; Surviving Prostate Cancer
By Michael Korda, Random House Paperback, 272 pages, 1997, ISBN 0679448446
This book seems to receive mixed reviews from Circlers. It was the first book I read after my diagnosis of prostate cancer, and I found it very informative. Mr. Korda underwent radical prostatectomy for his cancer, and paints a bleak picture of the process. That has been the source of criticism from some Circlers who have been through their own prostatectomies. I can personally recommend it to anyone contemplating prostate surgery.

Prostate Cancer; A Survivor's Guide
By Don Kaltenbach, with Tim Richards, Paperback, 274 pages, 1996, ISBN 0964008823
John C. Blasko, M.D. has written the forward.
Mr Kaltenbach elected radioactive seed implants for his own prostate cancer. He has written a well-rounded book describing the process, and discusses other options. I especially enjoyed his last chapter written for a man's spouse, "When Your Husband Has Prostate Cancer."

My Prostate And Me; Dealing With Prostate Cancer

By William Martin, Hardcover 246 pages, 1994,
ISBN 1569778884
Mr Martin relates his own experiences with prostate cancer.
It's well written and often humorous as he discusses the emo-
tional impact of prostate cancer and treatment options.
Includes an afterward by Peter Scardino, M.D., Chief of
Urology, Baylor College of Medicine.

***Coping With Prostate Cancer; A Guide to Living With
Prostate Cancer For You And Your Family.***
By Robert H. Phillips, Ph.D., Paperback, 291 pages, 1994
ISBN 0895295644
Robert Phillips is a practicing psychologist who offers "compassionate advice to those who must deal with prostate
cancer." His book begins with the basics of prostate cancer
and therapeutic options. He then moves quickly to the topics
of his expertise, the emotional states of depression, fear,
anger, anxiety, guilt, and even boredom, envy, loneliness, and
grief. He addresses ones' need for self care and lifestyle
changes in work and recreation. His last chapter addresses
one's significant other. "Living With Someone With Prostate
Cancer."

***Stress Management for Cancer Patients: A Self-Help Care
Manual***
By Morry Edwards, Ph.D., Paperback, 170+ pages, 2000
ISBN 0-9678801-1-4
This self-care manual is intended to help you learn skills and
implement effective strategies to ease the stress of cancer and
its treatment. Dr. Edwards offers a smorgasbord of techniques, ideas, and exercises to assist patients and family
members in strengthening emotional and mental well-being.
Advocating a holistic approach to health and wellness, the
author encourages patients to take an active role in their treatment. Includes a month-long journal.

***Love, Medicine & Miracles: Lessons Learned about Self-
Healing from a Surgeon's Experience with Exceptional
Patients***
By Bernie S. Siegel, M.D.
"My friend Nancy died some years ago of small cell lung
cancer, which metasticized to her brain. She said she had

been afraid of everything, but after reading this book she was no longer afraid of anthing."

***Contemporary Issues in Prostate Cancer:
A Nursing Perspective***
Edited By Jeanne Held-Warmkessel, MSN, RN, CS, AOCN, Fox Chase Cancer Center, Philadelphia, PA, Hardcover, 315 pages, 2000 ISBN 0-7637-1399-6
Comprehensive and up-to-date information on all aspects of risk factors, screening, diagnosis, and treatment options available in prostate cancer management. Excellent resource for accurate patient education and competent nursing care for men with prostate cancer. Very thorough!

CYBER-RESOURCES

Nancy Peress is an amazing woman. She tirelessly monitors *The Circle* every day. She has compiled a list of Internet resources for members of this support group, and mails it out every Friday—primarily for newcomers. It's a treasure trove of available information for anyone who can access the World Wide Web. She has given her consent to publish it here, with the hope that we can push back the curtain of confusion for those seeking help. Among the information listed here is an address for The Circle. This list is offered with a genuine invitation to join us.

MAILING LISTS

Note: Within a few minutes of subscribing to a mailing list, you should receive a confirmation message. Please follow the instructions exactly in order to activate your subscription.

Physician To Patient
The purpose of the p2p mailing list is to provide the prostate

cancer patient or other interested parties with information from physicians about the treatment of prostate cancer. This is a moderated list without the high volume normally associated with mailing lists or the frequent off-topic questions. To subscribe, send an email

> To: majordomo@prostatepointers.org
> Subject: (blank or a dash)
> subscribe p2p

The Circle
Support for wives, families, friends, and significant others of men with prostate cancer—and, of course, the men themselves. To subscribe, send an email:

> To: majordomo@prostatepointers.org
> Subject: (blank or a dash)
> subscribe circle

SeedPods
A mailing list for those interested in brachytherapy (radioactive seed implants) as a treatment for prostate cancer. To subscribe, send an email

> To: majordomo@prostatepointers.org
> Subject: (blank or a dash)
> subscribe seedpods

RP
A mailing list dedicated to the needs and concerns of radical prostatectomy patients. The sole purpose of this list is to narrowly focus on the concerns of those who have already had an RP or have selected RP as their treatment. To subscribe, go to: http://www.prostatepointers.org/mailman/listinfo

IceBalls
A mailing list offering information and support to those interested in cryosurgery for prostate cancer. To subscribe, send an email:

> To: majordomo@prostatepointers.org
> Subject: (blank or a dash)
> subscribe iceballs

CHB

CHB offers discussion and support for patients interested in any form of hormonal blockade. This includes: orchidectomy, medical hormonal blockade [lupron, flutamide, proscar, etc.] as well as food supplements such as PC-SPES. To subscribe, go to: http://www.prostatepointers.org/mailman/listinfo

EBRT

EBRT offers discussion and support for patients interested in any form of radiation therapy for prostate cancer. To subscribe, go to:
http://www.prostatepointers.org/mailman/listinfo

Prostate Cancer and Intimacy

PCAI is an unmoderated mailing list for frank and open discussion of the sexual issues surrounding PCa. To subscribe, send an email:
To: majordomo@prostatepointers.org
Subject: (blank or a dash)
subscribe pcai

Prostate Problems (PPML)

This is a medically intensive mailing list focusing primarily on the diagnosis and treatment of prostate cancer. To subscribe, send an email:
To: LISTSERV@listserv.acor.org
Subject: (blank or a dash)
subscribe prostate yourfirstname yourlastname
(example: subscribe prostate John Doe)
Or subscribe via the web:
http://www.acor.org/prostate.html

PC-SPES

This list is dedicated to promoting the most positive environment possible for the uninhibited exchange of information between patients who have chosen PC SPES as a treatment for their prostate cancer.

To subscribe to the main list, send an email to:

Majordomo@world.std.com with the following command
in the body of the message:
subscribe pc-spes <anybody@anywhere.com>
To subscribe to the digest version, send an email to:
Majordomo@world.std.com
with the following command in the message:
subscribe pc-spes-digest <anybody@anywhere.com>

Prostate Cancer Action Network
A forum for discussing important issues affecting the care
and treatment of prostate cancer survivors, and ways to bring
about needed change. To subscribe, go to:
http://www.prostatepointers.org/mailman/listinfo

Humor And Healing
HAH is a humor list for the online PCa community, more
intimate and friendly than the big Internet joke lists. To subscribe, go to:
http://www.prostatepointers.org/mailman/listinfo

Virtual Library
A library of documents available by email to those without
access to the World Wide Web: You may access the Virtual
Library by sending an email message:
  To: majordomo@prostatepointers.org
  Subject: (blank or a dash)
  info library
  This will return complete instructions for getting a current
  index of files and ordering the files you want.

PROSTATE CANCER WEB SITES

Prostate Pointers
http://www.prostatepointers.org/prostate

Prostate Cancer Profiler
http://www.cancerfacts.com/portal.asp?CancerTypeId=1

Prostate cancer acronyms and abbreviations:
http://www.prostatepointers.org/prostate/ed-pip/acronyms.html

Prostate cancer glossary of terms:
http://www.prostatepointers.org/prostate/ed-pip/glossary.html

Information provided by Nicholas Bruchovsky, MD
http://www.prostatepointers.org/bruchovsky

Information provided by Fernand Labrie, MD
http://www.prostatepointers.org/labrie

Information provided by Robert Leibowitz, MD
http://www.prostatepointers.org/prostate/leibowitz

Information provided by Charles Myers, MD
http://www.prostatepointers.org/cmyers

Information provided by Jonathan Oppenheimer, MD
http://www.prostatepointers.org/virtual_lab

A comprehensive list of papers by Steve Strum, MD
http://www.prostatepointers.org/strum/

Information provided by Israel Barken, MD
http://www.prostatepointers.org/barken

Physician to Patient
http://www.prostatepointers.org/p2p

SeedPods
http://www.prostatepointers.org/SeedPods/

IceBalls
http://www.prostatepointers.org/iceballs/

The Circle
http://www.prostatepointers.org/circle/

Organize your PC digest:
http://www.prostatepointers.org/rtrax/pcdigest.html

Tom Feeney's Watchful Waiting page:
http://www.prostatepointers.org/ww/

Search prostatepointers.org for information valuable to you! http://www.prostatepointers.org/search_form.html

The Education Center for Prostate Cancer Patients
http://www.ecpcp.org/main.html

Prostate Cancer Resource Guide
http://www.afud.org/pca/pcaindex.html

PPML archives:
http://listserv.acor.org/archives/prostate.html

The Wellness Web
http://wellweb.com

Prostate Cancer Dot Com
http://www.prostatecancer.com/

The Prostate Dictionary:
http://www.comed.com/Prostate/Glossary.html

The Prostate Cancer InfoLink:
http://www.comed.com/Prostate/index.html

Center for Prostate Disease Research
http://www.cpdr.org/

PC-SPES website:

http://www.pc-spes.com

PSA Rising Magazine
http://www.psa-rising.com

Prostate Cancer Action Network
http://www.prostatepointers.org/pcan/

Resources for making informed decisions about treatment options. http://www.cancerfacts.com

Powerful search engines and tools:
http://www.dogpile.com
http://www.northernlight.com/
http://www.copernic.com/
http://www.search.com/

PATIENTS HELPING PATIENTS WITH PROSTATE CANCER

Don Cooley is yet another survivor of prostate cancer, whose interest in medicine began as a medic in the Korean War. Don has lost two wives to cancer, and was able to use his medical knowledge in their care. When diagnosed with prostate cancer in 1997, he applied that medical experience in researching his own therapy. He chose brachytherapy combined with external beam radiation at the Radio Therapy Clinics of Georgia. Now almost three years later, his PSA continues to decline.

Don was one of the first survivors to begin telling his story on the Internet. He created a web site that began as a homespun place to relate to other survivors. Over the ensuing three years it has become a tour de force consisting of multiple discussion groups listing 1200 members and multiple informative web pages. Visit his web site at
htpp://www.cooleyville.com/cancer
or check out the related web sites below.

Prostate-Help Cancer (PHCa) Discussion Groups:
Following is a list of discussion groups/mailing lists to which patients and/or loved ones may subscribe. Most of these lists are unmoderated. A few have moderators, who select the messages to be posted, to keep the list on topic.

Prostate Help Discussion Group/Mailing List (PHML)
A general prostate cancer mailing list, covering all aspects of prostate cancer. Any questions about prostate cancer may be asked. Based on the "Team" concept of a cadre of knowledgeable "Team Prostate-Help" members helping each other.

> To: listserv@home.ease.lsoft.com
> Subject: blank
> Body of message: SUBSCRIBE PROSTATE-HELP

PHCa Brachytherapy (Seeds and HDR) Prostate Cancer Discussion Group (PHCa-Brachytherapy)
Serves those prostate cancer patients who are looking for help in their selection of treatment or the after effects of treatment. Heavy emphasis on studies and scientific research. Dedicated to all forms of Brachytherapy, including seed implant, HDR, EBRT and Hormonal therapy with Brachytherapy.

> Click to subscribe to PHCa-Brachytherapy

PHCa Advanced Prostate Cancer Discussion Group/Mailing List (PHCa-Advanced)
Serves patients and their loved ones who have had their primary treatment and the treatment has failed. Here you can post questions on what to do next, or inquire about advanced prostate cancer, various side effects, etc. Efforts are made to cover all advanced cancer treatments from hormonal ablation to chemo therapy and any other protocol used for patients whose primary treatment has failed.

> Click to subscribe to PHCa-Advanced

PHCa Alternatives Prostate Cancer Discussion Group/Mailing List (PHCa-Alternatives)
Designed to assist in a review of alternative and complimentary medicine, diet, etc. The aim is not to replace conventional treatments but to help patients discover alternatives and

complementary strategies that might assist or supplement treatment.

Click to subscribe to PHCa-Alternatives

PHCa-Watchful Waiting Discussion Group

Serves prostate cancer patients who would like information about Watchful Waiting and those who are presently doing so. It is not the intention of this list to promote Watchful Waiting but to help others understand what the advantages and pitfalls might be and to give them the benefit of the combined knowledge of the group.

Click to subscribe to PHCa-WW

PHCa Radiotherapy Clinic of Georgia Prostate-Help Group

Serves patients who have been and are being treated by Radiotherapy Clinic of Georgia (RCOG). Here they can discuss things that are involved with RCOG. A web site to track their progress and chart their PSA is available. It is a patient run group with no direct ties to RCOG.

Click to subscribe to RCOG-phg

Related web site: http://cooleyville.com/rcogalum

PHCa Newsletter

A Prostate-Help Newsletter list that will send a Newsletter on an "as needed" basis. The newsletter contains information that may be important in our fight with prostate cancer. Postings come from many sources, including studies and other posts. Designed for the delivery of information, not posting. Questions may be directed to cooleydd@pacbell.net

Click to subscribe to PHCa-Newsletter

Related web sites to all the above:
http://cooleyville.com/cancer
Email may be sent to Don Cooley at cooleydd@pacbell.net
Questions? Call Don Cooley at 408-268-6400

DOCTOR, I HAVE A FEW QUESTIONS?
(DON COOLEY & RUSS INGRAM)

Don Cooley worked with Russ Ingram to develop a list of questions, which he has posted on his website. Russ passed away December, 1998. This list is published with Don's permission and in memory of Russ Ingram.

This is an exhaustive list. As a physician, I would shudder if a patient appeared in my office and demanded answers to all of this! Think of this list as an outline of conversations you would like to have and pick those you feel a need to both ask and have answered.

SUGGESTED QUESTIONS

DIAGNOSIS

1. Has my cancer spread (metastasized) to other parts of my body?
2. What stage is my cancer?
3. Can you tell if this is a fast-growing type of prostate cancer, or a slow-growing type? (What is the Gleason score and ploidy type?)

TESTS

1. What tests will I have done?
2. When should I expect the results from these tests?
3. What will these tests tell me about my cancer?
4. How long after I have these tests will I know the results?
5. Who will call me with the results of these tests? Or, should I call to obtain the results?
6. If I need to get copies of my records, scans, X-rays, who can I contact?

PHYSICIAN

1. Did you consult with anyone before determining the diagnosis?

2. What will their role be in my treatment?

3. How many physicians will be involved in my care? Who are they? What are their roles?

4. Who will be the physician in charge of coordinating all the rest of my physicians?

5. What other health care professionals can I expect to be involved in my care?

6. Do you recommend surgery? If so, what are my options involving surgery?

7. Is nerve-sparing surgery possible in my ease?

8. What percentage (approximately) of the nerve-conserving surgeries you have done have been a success?

9. Would you give me the telephone number of two other patients?

TREATMENT

1. What is the standard treatment for my type of prostate cancer?

2. What is the prognosis for my type of prostate cancer with standard treatment?

3. Are there any other treatments that might be appropriate for my type of prostate cancer?

4. What treatment do you recommend? Based on what?

5. What are the risks or benefits of the treatment you are recommending?

6. Am I a good candidate for a radiation seed implant where the seeds are left in?

7. Am I a good candidate for a radiation seed implant where the seeds are inserted and removed?

8. Who would you recommend I talk to about the different treatments?

9. What doctors do you know who are experts at the seed implant radiation techniques?

10. What percentage of patients usually respond to this treatment?

11. How long does each treatment last?

12. How long will the entire course of therapy last?

13. How often will I be treated?

14. What type of results should I expect to see with the treatment?

15. Will there be tests during my treatment to determine if it is working?

16. Where will I receive my treatment?

17. How will I receive my treatment? Is it a pill? An injection?

18. What will it feel like to get treated?

19. Can someone accompany me to my treatment?

20. Can I drive to and from my appointments?

21. Can I stay alone after my treatments, or do I need to have someone stay with me?

22. Will I have to be in the hospital to get my treatments?

23. Who will administer my treatments?

24. How often, during treatment, will I see a physician? The nurse?

CLINICAL TRIALS

1. Are there any clinical trials or research being done on my type of prostate cancer?

2. Are you involved in clinical trials?

3. Would I be a candidate for clinical research if it is a treatment option for me?

4. Where can I find out more about research on prostate cancer?

5. Is there anyone else in the area that is involved in research that I might contact to discuss my prostate cancer?

6. What will happen if I decide not to be treated?

7. How quickly must I decide about my treatment?

ECONOMICS

1. How do I find out what portion of the treatment my insurance company will cover?

2. Is there someone in your of office (or facility) who assists patients with questions about insurance? Who would that be?

3. If my insurance does not pay for a particular treatment or medication that might be beneficial to me, will you choose an alternate treatment? What if it is less effective?

4. Do you have access to pharmaceutical patient assistance programs I could access if I cannot afford a particular medication or my insurance will not pay for a particular medication?

5. Who can I talk to about getting treatment if I do not have insurance?

SUPPORT

1. Do you have any literature that suggests ways to tell my family and friends of my illness?

2. Are you willing to speak with my wife (or other family members) about my prostate cancer and my treatment?

3. Are there support groups for prostate cancer?

4. For my family and friends?

5. Is there a social worker here I could talk to?

6. How do I access a dietitian if I have nutritional concerns or difficulties?

7. Do I need to be on a special diet?

8. If I can have sex after my treatment, will my partner be at risk in any way?

9. What type of precautions do I need to take?

10. Who do I call if I have an emergency medical situation during my treatment, or shortly afterwards?

11. What are the telephone numbers I should have in order to reach you? The nurse? The hospital?

SIDE EFFECTS

1. What are the side effects of this treatment?
   · Nausea
   · Vomiting
   · Hair loss
   · Low blood cell counts (anemia: low red-blood-cell count, neutropenia: low count of one type of white-blood cell, lowplatelets, etc.)
   · Diarrhea/constipation
   · Skin changes
   · Incontinence
   · Impotence
   · Pain
   · Sores along the digestive tract
   · Taste changes
   · Neuropathy (damage to nerves)
   · Slow heart beat
   · Irregular heart beat
   · Fatigue

2. When might these side effects occur?

3. Could these side effects be life-threatening?

4. How long will the side effects last?

5. What can/will be done to prevent these side effects or reduce their possibility?

6. When might these side effects occur?

7. Could these side effects be life-threatening?

8. How long will the side effects last?

SUPPORTIVE THERAPIES

1. What treatments are available to manage these side effects?

2. Are these support therapies available and appropriate for me?

3. What should I do if I have side effects?

4. Who do I call if I have severe side effects?

5. Will a reduction or delay reduce my chances of being cured?

6. Are there any medications I should not take while I'm going through treatment?

7. Are there any activities I should or should not do following treatment?